Eight Limbs of Yoga

–

The Structure and Pacing
of
Self-Directed Spiritual Practice

Yogani

From The AYP Enlightenment Series

AYP Publishing

For ordering information go to:

www.advancedyogapractices.com

Library of Congress Control Number: 2008901442

Published simultaneously in:

Nashville, Tennessee, U.S.A.
and
London, England, U.K.

This title is also available in eBook format – ISBN 978-0-9800522-9-9
(For Adobe Reader)

ISBN 978-0-9800522-8-2 (Paperback)

"Through practice of the limbs of Yoga,
whereby impurities are eliminated,
there arises enlightenment…"

Yoga Sutras of Patanjali – 2:28

Introduction

Centuries ago, a short scripture called the *Yoga Sutras* was written by the Indian sage, *Patanjali*, outlining the essential practices and experiences leading to the rise of human enlightenment. This concise scripture contains the famous *Eight Limbs of Yoga*, reflecting the natural spiritual capabilities within each of us, and the means for unfolding them.

The center of all spiritual progress is found within each human nervous system. When time-tested methods for stimulating the process of human spiritual transformation are applied in an integrated way, remarkable progress can occur within any cultural or religious setting. Now, anyone who has the desire can build a *self-directed* daily practice routine for the long term, leading to the steady cultivation of enlightenment in everyday life. This book details the overall structure, integration and pacing of yoga practices that have been presented in the previous extensive *Advanced Yoga Practices* (AYP) instructional writings.

The AYP Enlightenment Series is an endeavor to present the most effective methods of spiritual practice in a series of easy-to-read books that anyone can use to gain practical results immediately and over the long term. For centuries, many of these powerful practices have been shrouded in secrecy, mainly in an effort to preserve them. Now we find ourselves in the *information age*, and able to preserve knowledge for present and future generations like never before. The question remains: "How far can we go in effectively transmitting spiritual methods in writing?"

Since the beginning in 2003, the writings of AYP have been an experiment to see just how much can be conveyed, with much more detail included on practices than in the spiritual writings of the past. Can books provide us the specific means necessary to tread the path to enlightenment, or do we have to surrender at the feet of a *guru* to find our salvation? Well, clearly we must surrender to something, even if it is to our own innate potential to live a freer and happier life. If we are able to do that, and maintain regular practice, then books like this one can come alive and instruct us in the ways of human spiritual transformation. If the reader is ready and the book is worthy, amazing things can happen.

While one person's name is given as the author of this book, it is actually a distillation of the efforts of thousands of practitioners over thousands of years. This is one person's attempt to simplify and make practical the spiritual methods that many have demonstrated throughout history. All who have gone before have my deepest gratitude, as do the many I am privileged to be in touch with in the present who continue to practice with dedication and good results.

I hope you will find this book to be a useful resource as you travel along your chosen path.

Practice wisely, and enjoy!

Table of Contents

Chapter 1 – Eight Limbs of Yoga

Ever since our ancient ancestors gazed up to the heavens with a sense of wonder, there has been an intuitive knowing that we are something more than the physical mortal beings we appear to be.

But what? And how can we experience that in the fullest measure we are capable of?

This has been the riddle of humankind since our beginnings, and continues to be our greatest challenge in modern times. We have sailed the seas, traveled the skies, harnessed the atom, shrunk the world with instant communications, and flown into outer space. But have we realized the full inner potential of the human being? Not yet. Not on a mass scale.

Some may doubt that there is anything within us to realize. As the religious institutions of the world groan under the weight of ritual, superstition, politics and corruption, we may wonder if there is any truth to the idea that human beings are capable of the spiritual experiences and profound inner freedom promised in the world's scriptures since ancient times.

Yet, there have always been a few who have claimed from their own experience that human spiritual transformation is a fact, and attempted to show the way to it. Nearly everyone has sensed at one time or other the *something more* that lives within all of us. So we carry on with the quest for knowledge, and those who have seen through their inner door continue to teach the ways that are believed to facilitate such openings in all people.

While, for most of humankind, the world of spiritual endeavor has looked flat and foreboding for a long time, it is now becoming apparent to many that something wonderful lies just over the horizon. Those who have traveled there tell remarkable stories of abiding peace, ecstasy and outpouring divine love. There is even the prospect of finding the entire universe contained within ourselves. Indeed, the *final frontier* is within us!

While we may not be sure of all this, we can be sure of one thing. There is more that we can know, and we will know it in due course. The truth will set us free. Like knowledge in all fields of endeavor in this modern age of technology and information, spiritual knowledge is expanding rapidly. In the process, the ancient knowledge of spirit is finding application in new and efficient ways.

The Yoga Sutras of Patanjali

Centuries ago, a short scripture was written by the Indian sage, *Patanjali*, systematizing a range of practices for stimulating the natural capabilities inherent within every human nervous system, for purification and opening leading to direct realization of the condition we call *enlightenment*.

Patanjali's scripture is called the *Yoga Sutras* (meaning "stitches of union"), and it provides one the world's clearest summaries of the methods and experiences of human spiritual transformation.

The integrated practices described by Patanjali comprise the famous *Eight Limbs of Yoga*. This list is so complete in its coverage of human spiritual capabilities, and the means for unfolding them, that it can serve as a check-list for assessing the completeness of literally any spiritual path.

Patanjali's Eight Limbs of Yoga include:

- **Yama** (*restraints* – non-violence, truthfulness, non-stealing, preservation and cultivation of sexual energy, and non-covetousness)
- **Niyama** (*observances* – purity, contentment, spiritual intensity, study of spiritual knowledge and *Self*, and active surrender to the divine)
- **Asana** (postures and physical maneuvers)
- **Pranayama** (breathing techniques)
- **Pratyahara** (introversion of the senses)
- **Dharana** (systematic attention on an object)
- **Dhyana** (meditation – systematic dissolving of the object in consciousness)
- **Samadhi** (absorption in pure bliss consciousness)

There is an additional category of practice in the *Yoga Sutras* called **Samyama,** which employs the last three limbs of yoga at the same time. Patanjali discusses the practice of samyama with a dramatic flair in the *Yoga Sutras*, employing the phrase *supernormal powers* to describe the results, referring to the *siddhis and miracles* that are the incidental effects of samyama. In fact, samyama is a systematic method for stimulating an outpouring of *divine love* in daily life, which is the rise of *stillness in action* – the ongoing ecstatic union of inner and outer life. It is unending happiness, which is the greatest siddhi of them all.

Every system of yoga teaching has its own way of presenting the eight limbs of yoga. Sometimes, the limbs of yoga are taught in order, which is the traditional way – first learn the rules of conduct (yama and niyama), and then, if the student is considered worthy, the teacher may provide instruction for the more penetrating practices further down the list.

The eight limbs of yoga are so logical and easy to understand that virtually every teacher of yoga claims to be teaching them, which is true to one degree or another, because the eight limbs cover everything one can do in yoga. In this sense, they represent a complete road map, a blueprint and spiritual checklist of the various methods for opening the human nervous system to divine experience.

Taken together as an overall system, the eight limbs of yoga have been referred to as *ashtanga (eight-limbed) yoga* and *raja (royal) yoga*. But what is in a name? What we here call *Advanced Yoga Practices (AYP)* are the eight limbs too. So is any approach to human spiritual transformation, in whole or in part, including the systems of spiritual practice we find in the world's mainstream religions. If it has to do with human spiritual transformation, it is going to be found somewhere in the eight limbs. That is the beauty of the eight limbs. When we look at any spiritual teaching or religious tradition, using the eight limbs as a measuring rod, we see right away what is there, and what is not. The more enlightened traditions will have more of the limbs covered, and the less enlightened ones will have fewer limbs covered. This is not a sectarian consideration. It is a matter of what works, regardless of the cultural or religious clothing spiritual practices might happen to be wearing. Spiritual practice is like mathematics – not dependent on time, place or culture. One plus one will equal two everywhere. It is cause and effect.

The eight limbs of yoga capture the whole of spiritual cause and effect with elegant simplicity.

As mentioned, traditionally, the eight limbs have been taken in sequence. The rationale has been that people have to learn to behave themselves and prepare through strict codes of conduct before they can begin doing more direct spiritual practices. Once they know how to behave rightly, they can begin with the body (asanas), and, later, work their way on through the breath (pranayama), and, finally, be ready for focused attention (dharana), meditation (dhyana), and pure bliss consciousness (samadhi). With a traditional approach like this it can be a long road to travel, especially if the teacher holds his or her students to the highest standards of performance each step along the way. Even Patanjali had this sequence of practice in mind when he wrote the yoga sutras.

That part of it (learning the eight limbs in sequence over a long period) doesn't work very well in modern times, where the emphasis is on optimizing causes and effects in the most efficient manner. It makes sense to streamline the methods of yoga in time, because we are all working with a limited life-span, with time being at a premium. Over the past century, the urgency for more effective applications of practice has become widely recognized in the yoga community, and many innovations in teaching have occurred. In the time of Patanjali, perhaps it was not so easy to be jump-starting people with advanced practices like deep meditation and spinal breathing pranayama the way it is routinely done today. These changes represent progress.

Over the years, different teachers have jumped directly into the eight limbs in different places. Some start with asanas, and others with pranayama. Some focus first on devotion and then jump to meditation, or something else. Some jump straight into meditation, and then work their way back through the limbs. Interestingly, such "highest first" approaches lead to spiritual conduct (yama and niyama) rising as an effect of inner purification and opening, rather than being used as a primary cause through strict rules of conduct, which can be very inefficient.

The strategy in the *AYP writings* is along the lines of the latter *highest first* approach. Here we begin with deep meditation, and then move into pranayama, physical techniques, samyama, and so on, cultivating the primary engine of bhakti (spiritual desire) all the way through. In this book we will be discussing the overall process of building and managing our practice routine along these lines.

One thing everyone who does yoga for a while has found is that the limbs of yoga are connected. Meaning, if we start in one limb, the other limbs will be affected. As we purify and open from within, we will eventually be drawn into all of the limbs.

It is common for new meditators to become voracious spiritual readers (a niyama – study), lean toward a purer diet (a niyama – purity), and feel more sensitive about the wellbeing of others (a yama – non-harming).

In fact the best way to achieve progress in yama and niyama is by going straight to samadhi (pure bliss consciousness – inner silence) with deep meditation. Then harmonious behavior comes naturally from inside, rather than having to be enforced from outside. These results are indicators of the *connectedness of yoga*. It occurs on all levels of practice. Sometimes it is called *grace*, because spiritual blessings seem to come out of nowhere. In truth, such blessings are being telegraphed through us via spiritual conductivity rising in our nervous system from something we did somewhere on the eight-limbed tree of yoga.

Even the sincere heart-felt inquiry, "Is there something more than this?" is a powerful yoga practice. It is found in niyama – it is bhakti, active surrender to our chosen highest ideal.

As we advance in our yoga practices, this conductivity in the nervous system becomes ecstatic. Then we call it *ecstatic conductivity* (also referred to as *kundalini*). When the conductivity within us becomes ecstatic, we are really getting connected through the limbs of yoga – here, there, and everywhere.

If we engage in effective practices in multiple limbs, built up in a systematic step-by-step way, then our nervous system will be purifying and opening most rapidly. This is an important principle that is at the core of the AYP approach – using a broad integrated system of effective practices, having the option of working through as many limbs as possible in a self-directed way, at our own speed.

In this way the focus of spiritual development moves naturally from external institutions and teachers to the place where the transformation and spiritual experience are actually occurring, within each person. This is the rightful destiny of all people, and it is time for each of us to claim it as our own. The sooner we do, the sooner we will be on our way.

It has long been thought that spiritual wisdom is most relevant when it is ancient, coming through mysterious preceptors, and somehow divorced from our present reality. The truth is that spiritual knowledge is totally ancient and totally modern – totally human in the here and now, and capable of coming alive within every one of us. This is why in the *AYP writings*, we often say, "The guru is in you."

Yoga and the Human Nervous System

While yoga is a fascinating subject to read about, ponder and discuss, the real benefits come from direct application of its methods. Yoga is regarded to be a philosophy in India, and this is really a misnomer. It is much more than that. Yoga is a system of methods designed to promote the natural process of human spiritual transformation on the individual level.

In modern times, yoga is often thought to mean physical postures, *asanas*, which is but one of the eight limbs. A quick review of the *Yoga Sutras of Patanjali* reveals that yoga covers a much broader field than postures, encompassing multiple tools that take advantage of multiple capabilities for transformation inherent within the human nervous system.

Yoga means *union* – union of the inner and outer qualities of life. This is more than a philosophy. It is a living reality, cultivated through a variety of methods applied systematically on a daily basis. All the limbs of yoga are connected within us.

In fact, <u>all of yoga is a product of the human nervous system</u>. Not the other way around, as we sometimes may tend to think. What has for so long been regarded to be an external knowledge is actually an internal knowledge that is far more accessible to us than is commonly believed. As soon as we understand that our spiritual possibilities are an internal process rather than an external one, then a profound shift in our development will begin to happen. On the individual level the shift can be quite rapid. And it can encompass an entire society as radiant energy goes out, leading to a rise in intuitive understanding and increased use of spiritual practices among the people. In this way, all of humankind can be uplifted.

It took a while for people to believe that the world is round instead of flat, and that the sun is the center of the solar system instead of the earth. It took some proof. Then almost everyone believed, and the rush was on to derive the benefits of the new knowledge, the new paradigm.

Now it is time for us to come to grips with the fact that the human nervous system is the center of all spiritual experience and of all divine bliss. That is your nervous system, the one you are sitting in right now. The doorway to the infinite is that close within us. The sooner we get used to the idea that each of us is a direct gateway to the divine, the better it will be for everyone. As with the acceptance of any knowledge, it takes some proof. In this case, the proof is in each of us. We don't have to rely on others for proof for very long. Open a few doors here and there by doing some effective yoga practices and we will soon see what we are. Then the rush will be on to open it all up. A new paradigm is born!

What are the benefits of the knowledge of yoga and its effective application? It is a natural transformation to a higher functioning of our nervous system that brings us more peace, creativity, energy and good health in daily living. We find ourselves to be more at *One* with the world, and more able to move within it in ways that benefit both ourselves and others. Fear and suffering become much less, no matter how much turmoil there may be in outer life. We become at *One* with the infinite ocean of life upon which all events in time and space are but waves upon the surface. The changes of life continue to come and go like the waves. Within, we remain steady, just as the depths of the ocean are. This is the fruit of yoga – not an idea, belief or philosophy, but a state of being, a living experience.

Nothing is new, you know. Our ancient ancestors heard of these things. Much of it was written down, and there have always been wise people who taught methods for living the truth residing within everyone. But communications were poor, life was often perilous, and people lived in so much fear and superstition. It is different now. We can find almost any information we want. There are so many doors of knowledge opening to everyone. The old wisdom is becoming new again, and expanding in its practical utilization. The human nervous system has not changed over the centuries. It has been waiting patiently, like a treasure chest longing to be opened. It is time.

Patanjali's Yoga Sutras, written centuries ago, is one of the greatest scriptures of all time. Not only does it tell us what we are, but it also tells us how the doors of the nervous system can be opened. It clearly describes the relationships between the natural principles of purification and opening that exist within us.

In the *AYP Enlightenment Series*, we have been traveling through the eight limbs in an order that expedites human spiritual transformation in ways that also take into account the maintenance of comfort and safety. Keep in mind that Patanjali was describing the inner workings of the human nervous system. The nervous system is what it is, and no one defines how it works. We can only do our best to describe it, understand its underlying principles, find the control levers to open it, and use them to our best advantage in the times we live in.

Once we know the practices of yoga, and can apply them in an effective integrated way, the rest is automatic. The primary purpose of intellectual understanding of spiritual matters (the dissection of processes into named elements/limbs) is to develop the means and confidence in what we are doing so we will be motivated to continue daily practices. Other than for that purpose, we don't need to know much about the inner workings. It is all going on out of sight. Like the engine in a car, it is under the hood. We just press on the gas pedal and away we go. It is that simple. So simple that many have missed it for thousands of years. It is time for everyone to be informed about what we all have – this human nervous system, this gateway to the divine that can be easily opened if we know where the simple controls are.

Yoga has been called a *science* before, often by traditionalists attempting to appeal to the modern mind as they promote inflexible by-rote methods. Yoga can be a real science if it becomes attuned to natural phenomena and the optimization of causes and effects in practice. This involves taking preserved knowledge, like the *Yoga Sutras*, and building on it with practical applications geared toward results rather than adherence to fixed approaches. The forward march of applied knowledge is a function of practices and the resulting experiences in the present, and making adjustments as necessary to achieve maximum progress with comfort and safety.

Real yoga science is interested in reliable results that anyone can produce using the most efficient methods, and is always looking for better ways to utilize natural principles operating in the nervous system to open to the infinite within.

Let's now look more closely at our inherent spiritual capabilities, and how the practices of yoga can be systematically used to awaken them.

14   – Eight Limbs of Yoga

Chapter 2 – The Structure of Practices

Spiritual practices find their origin in the human neurobiology, the vehicle of all our experience. Practices act to stimulate natural principles operating within the human being, which to a degree are seen to be automatic once the processes of transformation are underway. To the extent the vehicle of experience (our body/mind) can be stimulated to purify and open to express the reality within, then this is the way to *enlightenment*. Because of the intimate connection between spiritual methods and the human organism, the field of yoga, which covers the broad range of all spiritual practices, can be said to be at least as complex as any of the modern sciences relating to human functioning.

But this does not imply the impossibility of applying simple means for taking practical advantage of the complex inner workings of nature. We see this occurring all around us – the mastery of unseen principles with easy-to-use methodologies, or *control levers*. Consider the examples of modern aviation, biotechnology, computers, telecommunications, and a host of other advanced applied sciences. We call these fields *advanced*. Yet, how difficult is it to operate a cell phone, a computer, or walk onto an airplane and travel across the continent in a few hours? These applications of complex principles in nature are *advanced* <u>because</u> they have been simplified for practical application.

This is what we mean when we say *advanced yoga practices*. The practices will only be advanced if they are easy to use while stimulating complex processes within us for the benefit of our spiritual evolution. If they do, then they are advanced. If they do not, or can be made even simpler and more effective, then we will continue to seek out better ways for promoting the process of human spiritual transformation. That is the never-ending forward march of applied knowledge. It is the same in yoga as in any other field.

But yoga has been around for thousands of years, and has been well documented. What then could there possibly be that can be improved upon? Well, for a number of reasons, yoga has not been applied to the point where the whole of humanity has been able to benefit, so the evolution in knowledge must go on in modern times. It is a matter of simplifying the methods further, while increasing effectiveness, and providing easy access for everyone who wants to open to spiritual realization within themselves.

Simplification does not mean ignoring the basic realities of human spiritual transformation. There is a tendency we all have to seek what has been called a *magic bullet* solution. Do this one thing and all things will be solved. This is going to the opposite extreme on the complexity scale – from too complicated and ineffective to too simple and ineffective. We cannot drive a car with only a steering wheel. We also need a gas pedal and a brake. On the other hand, we cannot drive a car if we have to manually fire the spark plugs, pump the oil and coolant, manage the electrical system, and run all the other complex processes going on under the hood of the car. If the car is well-designed and built, the basic controls for steering, accelerating and braking are all we need. For those who are really into driving, then a manual gear shift and clutch can be added. That is pretty much the limit of what most of us can manage while driving a car.

Yoga is like this too. There are a number of key controls that address inner processes in the body/mind. If we attend to these efficiently, then there will be inner purification and opening, a gradual rise of spiritual experience, and steady progress toward enlightenment. If we fixate on a single yoga practice, we will find something lacking sooner or later. And if we try to do too many practices, we can become overwhelmed and likely experience confusing and unmanageable results.

So, what we are looking for here is a process of developing a balanced optimization of the main controls. We will begin with a review of our inner capabilities for making the journey of human spiritual transformation. Then we will lay out the most effective tools, found throughout the eight limbs of yoga. And finally we will apply the tools in a logical manner for best results, leaning toward neither the overly simplified approach nor the overly complex approach. For each of us the daily practice routine will be a bit different, depending on our spiritual desire and personal inclinations. But for most of us there is a range of practices that constitutes the center – the middle way. That is what we will aim for here, the middle way for each of us.

Our Inherent Spiritual Capabilities

Since the human nervous system is the center of all spiritual practice and the vehicle by which all spiritual progress is achieved, we will review our inherent spiritual capabilities and abilities, and see how these can lead to the application of effective spiritual practices covered in the eight limbs of yoga. We will also see how the practices that are covered in the eight limbs, and in the instructional writings of AYP, are as much a manifestation of our internal evolutionary impulses as a teaching that may happen to come to us from the outside.

Indeed, when approached rightly, the eight limbs of yoga are a reminder and a confirmation of what we have within us and intuitively know about ourselves already. This is borne out as we engage in practices, when the phenomenon of automatic yoga occurs – elements of yoga practice occurring automatically that we may not have been instructed in, or even ever heard of.

The *AYP writings* already cover a large number of practices in detail. Here we are summarizing the overall structure and pacing of a cohesive practice routine we can build using all the pieces. Does this mean there is nothing more to add to the system in the way of practices? We will likely never get to the stage of having a perfect system of practices, because the field of human spiritual transformation is vast, and there is much room for discovery and improvement. There are many complementary and integrative applications of practice that can be devised, and it is expected that research will continue for ongoing optimization of practices on the basis of causes and effects. It is the way of science.

With the knowledge and practices that are being applied now, so much purification and opening deep in our nervous system can be achieved that everything else that is necessary for enlightenment will come automatically through the connectedness of yoga. That is the objective of the *AYP writings* – to provide the essential means to stimulate the nervous system to purify and open itself, which it is very inclined to do when given the opportunity. Once the ball gets rolling, many aspects of our natural inclination toward human spiritual transformation will kick in. The goal here is to assist everyone to become self-sufficient in yoga like that.

Fundamental Principles and Natural Abilities

At the core of our spiritual development are the natural abilities contained within all of us, which only need some stimulation to move us toward conscious inner openings to the infinite. These abilities are rooted in several fundamental principles that are inherent in our nervous system. We are all designed and built to experience unending divine ecstatic bliss!

The fundamental principles of human spiritual transformation are simple enough. There are five of them, and they will be obvious to anyone who has considered their spiritual possibilities:

- **Attraction** – To truth and/or God, expressed as desire – It is Love.

- **Purification and Opening** – A process every human nervous system is naturally inclined to go through.

- **Inner Silence** – Pure bliss consciousness, our native state that shines through our nervous system as purification and opening occur.

- **Ecstasy** – Experienced when our nervous system is stimulated by the awakening of our inner life-force.

- **Union** – our transformation to a permanent state of radiating compassionate unity, the fruition of the merging of our inner silence and ecstasy – It is Love.

These five fundamental principles of enlightenment begin with love and end with love. Love is attraction manifesting as the force of desire and devotion to our highest ideal (bhakti), leading us through the process of human spiritual transformation. In that, we undergo the purification and opening of our nervous system, which reveals the principles of inner silence and ecstatic conductivity in us, and their merging in an outpouring of divine love and unity.

To accomplish this, we will be inspired to employ spiritual methods, which take advantage of natural abilities contained within us that are associated with the fundamental principles. Let's list those abilities now:

1. The ability that desire, consistently applied toward an objective, has to move our inner and outer expressions of energy (life-force) in ways that fundamentally change our experience of life.

2. The ability our mind has to move naturally beyond itself toward stillness. This is awareness without any objects – also called inner silence, or pure bliss consciousness.

3. The ability of the mind to effortlessly refine the thought of a sound (a mantra), naturally bringing the mind to stillness over and over again. Certain sounds resonate with our nervous system. These sounds can be used selectively to stimulate the nervous system toward an orderly transformation.

4. The mind-body connection that enables naturally cultivated stillness of mind to induce stillness of our body, metabolism, and breath. This happens through the connectedness of yoga, experienced in many ways through our nervous system.

5. The ability of our nervous system to naturally sustain the quality of stillness, our silent blissful inner consciousness, even when it is not being cultivated. This is called a state of the *silent witness*, among other things.

6. The ability of restraint and regulation of breath to stimulate the flow of life-force in the nervous system, producing a sensation of relaxation and the sensation of ecstasy in the body.

7. The ability of inner silence and the flow of life-force in the body to remove obstructions lodged deep in our nervous system, purifying and opening our awareness gradually to an expanding experience of inner peace, creative energy, happiness, and love.

8. The ability of restraint and regulation of breath to awaken the vast storehouse of life-force located in our pelvic region – sexual energy that is drawn upward in our nervous system to compensate for a reduced intake of oxygen when the breath is gently restrained.

9. The ability of attention to influence the flow of the life-force in the body, especially when combined with restraint and regulation of breath.

10. The ability of certain nerves and nerve plexuses to be stimulated physically to enhance and direct the flow of life-force in the body.

11. The ability of the neurobiology in the center and front of the head (the third eye) to connect with and direct (control) the neurobiology near the base of the spine and the vast storehouse of life-force (sexual energy) in that region.

12. The ability of the nerve in the center of the spine to conduct the life-force and ecstatic energy between the pelvic region and the third eye. This is called the spinal nerve (sushumna).

13. The ability of the spinal nerve to radiate life-force and ecstatic energy throughout the entire body and beyond, enlivening every aspect of the higher neurobiology within us and the environment around us in a smooth and orderly way. This is the rise of ecstatic radiance, or kundalini.

14. The ability of the nervous system to amplify the power of a thought when the thought is released deep in inner silence, yielding great purifying effects in the body and surrounding environment.

15. The ability of inner silence and ecstatic energy to merge and be sustained as *One* self-conscious presence in our nervous system. This is experienced as ecstatic bliss. Through natural inquiry in stillness, we come to know this as the expression of our divine *Self*.

16. The ability of ecstatic bliss to flow out from us to our surroundings as divine love. Then we find our

Self in the form of all we encounter. This is the natural flowering of divine love in service to all beings.

All of these abilities exist in us, and only need some nudging to begin to manifest changes in how our nervous system is functioning. With a full range of yoga practices (or even just a few essential ones), we can do a lot of nudging, stimulating every natural ability we have that can move us along the path of human spiritual transformation.

Everyone reacts a little differently to the processes of stimulation through yoga practices, due to the differences we each have in the structure of inner obstructions that are to be steadily and safely dissolved. We all can make the journey of transformation through yoga. It is only a matter of managing the conduct of our practices. This we call, *self-directed practice*, which involves implementing a strategy for building a progressive and safe daily practice routine. This is done step-by-step, as discussed in the next chapter.

To do this we draw from a wide range of practices that stimulate the activation of the abilities listed above, bringing to our conscious experience the fulfillment of the five fundamental principles.

An Inventory of Practices

We have talked about fundamental principles and our inherent abilities for human spiritual transformation. Now, how do we put all of that into motion? Clearly, the practices we use, how we apply them, and what the results are in our daily life are where the rubber meets the road.

Spiritual practices have been under development and applied for thousands of years, beginning with the methods used by our ancient ancestors who lived close to the land as hunter/gatherers and farmers. Ancient rites and rituals often formed the heart of spiritual practice in those days, with the hope of achieving a better life in harmony with nature. Over time, methods were refined to accommodate the occurrences within the human nervous system itself, and the focus gradually turned inward. The *Yoga Sutras of Patanjali* represent one of the pinnacles of understanding from ancient times. Many of the ancient scriptures in use today reflect similar understandings formed by our ancestors, based on the experiences of a few. Now it is time for us to expand on the ancient knowledge, based on the experiences of the many.

So, let's look at an inventory of practices reflecting what has been presented in the instructional writings of AYP. These have been assembled over the years by weighing the effectiveness of individual practices. And, more importantly, by weighing the effectiveness of the *integration* of practices. The practices listed as a whole do not represent any one tradition. They do represent the full range of the *Eight Limbs of Yoga*, not by necessity, but by virtue of their effectiveness in actual practice. Both the practices and the eight limbs are derived from the characteristics of the nervous system and its natural abilities to undergo the process of human spiritual transformation.

These descriptions of practices are not intended to be instructions for the practices, which can be found in the rest of the *AYP writings*. We are listing these here to prepare for the broader task of assembling a daily practice routine in a step-by-step fashion. By the time you have completed this book, it is hoped you will have a good feel for the overall structure and pacing of *self-directed spiritual practice*.

Here is our inventory of practices, the building blocks we will be using throughout the rest of this book:

1. **Bhakti** – cultivation of desire for our highest chosen ideal (love of truth and/or God in the heart), leading to daily practices. Bhakti/desire is the engine that drives all yoga practices. We accomplish it by favoring our chosen highest ideal (ishta), using this to systematically redirect our desires and emotions, whether they are positive or negative. In this way, a huge momentum driving us toward enlightenment is created within us and around us. Then everything we need to progress on our journey is drawn to us magnetically, including the willpower to engage in daily yoga practices for as long as it takes to complete our journey.

2. **Deep Meditation** with the mantra *I AM* (AYAM), plus several mantra enhancements added over time. Deep meditation involves easily favoring

the mantra to bring the mind (and body) to stillness over and over again twice-daily, stimulating deep purification in our nervous system, and yielding permanent blissful inner silence.

3. **Spinal Breathing Pranayama** – the primary practice for awakening and balancing the life-force in the spinal nerve between the third eye (brow) and root (perineum). It is the rise of ecstatic conductivity and radiance. This is also called the awakening of *kundalini*. Spinal breathing can be enhanced through a series of add-ons to practice, increasing the stimulation of the life-force in the spinal nerve.

4. **Mulabandha/Asvini** – manipulations using the anal sphincter and other muscles in the lower pelvic region to awaken the life-force (kundalini) at the root.

5. **Sambhavi Mudra** – a means for producing direct physical stimulation of the neurological mechanisms of the third eye in the head, involving gently raising and centering of the eyes toward the point between the eyebrows, and slightly furrowing the brow. Controlled and stable stimulation of kundalini at the root and throughout the nervous system is achieved in this way.

6. **Asanas (postures)** – systematic bending and stretching of the body that is a natural complement to spinal breathing pranayama and deep meditation. Asanas help cultivate and purify the nervous system, facilitating the rise of abiding inner silence and ecstatic conductivity in the body.

7. **Siddhasana** – a powerful way of sitting during practices for awakening ecstatic kundalini at the root, applying the principle of preservation and cultivation of sexual energy. The heel is placed at the perineum during spinal breathing and deep meditation, and constant pre-orgasmic stimulation of sexual energy is achieved. Over time, the entire nervous system is illuminated by this procedure when effectively and comfortably integrated with sitting practices.

8. **Yoni Mudra Kumbhaka** – a powerful practice (used sparingly) that helps open the third eye with air pressure in the nasal passages and sinuses, and awakening the life-force (kundalini) in the entire nervous system. This is accomplished through breath retention (kumbhaka) and an array of mudras and bandhas that, all together, constitute yoni mudra kumbhaka.

9. **Tantric Sexual Relations** (the holdback method, plus additional practices) – similar to the dynamics of siddhasana and used during normal sexual relations with or without a partner,

applying the principle of preservation and cultivation of sexual energy. When utilized in addition to daily sitting practices, tantric sexual methods are a powerful additional means for enlivening and distributing the life-force (kundalini) throughout the body.

10. **Kechari Mudra** (several stages) – this is gradually over time raising the tip of the tongue upward to (1) the roof of the mouth where the hard and soft palates meet, (2) above the soft palate to the spiritually erogenous rear edge of the nasal septum, (3) to the top of the nasal pharynx cavity, and (4) to the point between the eyebrows alternating through the spiritually sensitive nasal passages from the inside. Entering stage 2 kechari is a dramatic transition, especially when in relationship with ecstatic conductivity resulting from the application of an integration of yoga practices. Kechari is an important stimulator of an already stirring kundalini (indicated by an ecstatic sensitivity in the septum), playing an important role in the establishment of permanent body-wide ecstatic conductivity and radiance.

11. **Uddiyana Bandha and Nauli** – stimulating the upward movement of ecstatic energy, particularly via the digestive system, using the diaphragm and abdominal muscles after the breath is expelled. Nauli involves twirling the abdominal muscles, which stimulates the ecstatic neurobiology in and around the gastrointestinal tract.

12. **Dynamic Jalandhara (chin pump)**, with or without kumbhaka (breath retention). This is rotating the head while systematically dropping the chin toward the hollow of the throat with each rotation, stimulating ecstatic energies between the heart and head, and throughout the body.

13. **Samyama** – the process of initiating and releasing particular thoughts (sutras) deep within our inner silence, producing powerful purifying effects throughout the nervous system and beyond. The effects can manifest as so-called *supernormal powers*, which are also called *siddhis or miracles*. Samyama is performed for spiritual purification and the realization of life as an unending flow of *stillness in action*. There are several kinds of samyama: core samyama practice, cosmic samyama (yoga nidra), asana samyama, prayer samyama, and the cultivated habit of utilizing samyama to enhance many aspects of daily life.

14. **Spinal Bastrika Pranayama** – rapid breathing in the spinal nerve between the third eye (brow) and root (perineum), which accelerates the purification of the spinal nerve, and the entire nervous system. Bastrika can also be targeted to particular areas of resistance in the spinal nerve.

15. **Diet and Shatkarmas** (cleansing techniques) – these are modes of conduct (niyamas) for purifying the body and enhancing stillness and

ecstatic energy flow through the nervous system. Digestion plays a key role in the rise of ecstasy in the neurobiology, producing refined substances that illuminate the entire body and beyond. It has long been known that a light and nutritious diet will aid in spiritual development, as will reduced reliance on alcohol, tobacco and recreational drugs. Occasional fasting can also aid with inner purification and opening, as will the moderate use of amaroli (urine therapy). Further spiritual benefits can be gained through the use of cleansing methods (shatkarmas) for the gastrointestinal tract, nasal passages and sinuses. For best effectiveness, these methods rely on the application of a range of daily yoga practices, which cultivate inner silence and ecstatic conductivity in the nervous system. As we advance in deep meditation, we may naturally be drawn to these methods through the connectedness of yoga within us.

16. **Self-Inquiry** (recognition of our non-dual *Self*) – a natural questioning arising during daily activity, leading inevitably to the recognition of our essential nature – the absolute stillness of pure bliss consciousness, the unifying ground state of all existence. It may begin with the question, "Who am I?" Self-inquiry is often associated with our original spiritual desire (bhakti), and later on, aids us as we near the fruition of enlightenment. The relationship of our inquiry into reality will depend on the intensity of our bhakti and the

cultivation of inner silence (the witness) through deep meditation. Before then, self-inquiry will be little more than a mental exercise, and often a confusing and frustrating one, because the mind cannot deliver enlightenment. We must go beyond the mind. Enlightenment is not an idea. It is a condition of the nervous system, yielding perception of all inner and outer experiences (including thinking) from the perspective of inner silence, our silent witness, our divine *Self*.

17. **Karma Yoga** (loving service to others) – a natural practice that we find emerging in everyday living, a result of increasing inner silence, ecstatic radiance and the outward flow of divine love. This is due to the purification and opening of the nervous system from yoga practices. It is the rise of our natural state of being – abiding inner silence and an endless overflowing of ecstatic bliss and divine love. This is the great truth that is inherent in everyone – the reality of divine love. As we become advanced in yoga, this becomes crystal clear. For some it is known right from the very first sitting in deep meditation. All practices are but stepping stones leading us from our initial desire for fulfillment (bhakti) through the necessary purification and opening to the final expression of *That* in karma yoga, doing for others as we would do for ourselves, because we recognize others to be expressions of our own *Self*.

The above practices are the core methods of yoga utilized in the AYP system, based on practical application of our inherent spiritual capabilities for human spiritual transformation that have been discussed previously. In the next chapter we will discuss how these practices can be used to build an effective daily routine of practices that is compatible with a busy life in the world. In fact, the routine will be structured in a way that will automatically utilize our everyday activities as spiritual practice, without us having to give it a second thought.

Before we get into building the practice routine, we will take a look at the overall journey we will be taking.

The Journey of Purification and Opening

Suppose we want to begin doing some of the practices just listed. Say we have a strong desire for personal growth, and decide to undertake daily deep meditation. What will happen?

Our experience can be practically anything, ranging from little to nothing noticed going on, to some inner silence, to the sensation of mountains moving inside us. It can be all of these, occurring at different times over months and years of our daily practice. Our expectations will not be a cause in what happens, except as we expect to stay regular in our daily sittings, and abide by the procedure of our practice. Beyond that, expectations can become an impediment, a distraction. So it is good to just do our daily practice and go about our business in normal activities. Normal activity during the day is also important, as it plays an essential role in stabilizing what we are gaining in our meditation practice.

Once we undertake daily deep meditation, and later add other practices in a step-by-step fashion, we have embarked on a journey of purification and opening. All of our experiences will be related to that. As we cultivate inner silence (samadhi), a vast and complex process will be stimulated within us that can be described as *stillness in action*. As we go deep within, we stimulate and awaken a cosmic force which is the essence of our being. This will express within us and in our daily life in a multitude of ways. It is a natural process of awakening we are stimulating, one where our nervous system is drawn to a much higher level of functioning. In doing so, long time impurities and obstructions within us will automatically be dissolved. The symptoms of the purification process will appear in thoughts, feelings and physical manifestations. This is what the journey is about – purification and opening. It is important for us to understand this, since much of what we are doing on our path has to do with managing this process for maximum progress with comfort and safety. If we do not do this, then excessive symptoms of purification and opening can occur, leading to discomforts of various kinds and a corresponding loss of motivation to continue with daily practices.

Imagine a pipe (our nervous system) that is pretty clogged up, so it does not carry as much water (pure bliss consciousness) as it could. So we hook the pipe up to a powerful water supply (deep meditation) and the flow through the pipe is increased, but not without some resistance to the new level of flow and quite a lot of muck will be coming out the other end of the pipe as it is being cleaned out. This is the story of purification and opening of our nervous system as the process of human spiritual transformation progresses over time. And it does take some time. Contrary to what some may say, enlightenment is not an overnight event. While levels of realization may seem sudden, there are many of them to go through and that takes time in daily practices and ongoing regulation of practices to facilitate the process of purification and opening. We call it *self-pacing*.

Another way to look at this process, reflecting the changing quality of our experience as we advance, is the analogy of the sun and the clouds in the sky. As we progress with deep meditation and other spiritual practices, we will have glimpses of our own inner silence, which can take on the quality of shining radiance. Maybe we will just feel more clear for a while, more in stillness, or perhaps we will actually feel luminous from within. Then, just as the inner light came, it may go for a while, much the way the sun may disappear for a while when a cloud passes before it on a lovely day. With our practices, we have been clearing the clouds that block our inner light, our inner sun. And, and in time, the clouds will become very few and far between, and we will become a much purer vehicle of the light. This is how our activities in our normal daily life become elevated in many ways. The more inner silence we find ourselves to be, the fewer obstructions will be passing before our inner light, and the more we will be living an illumined life.

These two analogies, the pipe and the sunny sky, provide an idea about how the process of purification and opening will progress over time as we undertake and continue our self-directed spiritual practices. At times, we may feel that purification and opening are rather thick and mucky, like the pipe being flushed out with water. At other times, we may feel quite light and bright, like a sunny day, with the only breaks being a few wispy clouds passing before our vision, and then they are gone again. There are many levels of experience in the overall process of purification and opening as we move along on our path to enlightenment. It is like a long car journey with lots of scenery we pass by on the way. Some of the scenery may be beautiful, and other scenery not so beautiful. Whatever the scenery is like, we keep driving ahead at a good pace, without going too fast as we pass through the inevitable rough patches. Neither do we stop traveling to follow the calls of the exotic spiritual experiences we are likely to encounter. These are part of the scenery too. We enjoy the ride, but also carry on to our destination of abiding inner silence, ecstatic bliss, outpouring divine love and unity.

Now we will take a closer look at the art of developing a self-directed routine of practices that is best suited for our individual needs. With good practical information on effective practices and their use in hand, and steadily increasing first hand experience, who will be better qualified to advise us on how to do this than us?

Chapter 3 – Self-Directed Practice

We have reviewed the broad structure of integrated practices in the *Eight Limbs of Yoga* and delved into the specifics of what these practices are and how they relate to our inherent capabilities for undergoing the process of human spiritual transformation. We have also developed an idea about the journey of purification and opening that spiritual practices will take us on. The next step is to put it all together into a form that will be suitable for building a long term daily practice routine that is compatible with our particular nature and circumstances. It is time for us to take charge, and use what has been provided. We call it *self-directed spiritual practice*.

As we will see, there are several parts to self-directed practice – our daily sitting practices and other less structured practices we may choose to undertake during our normal daily activities. The objective is to find a balance that enlivens our life in a healthy way, without weighing us down with an excess of spiritual methods and concerns. A spiritual life is a happy life, unfettered by the burdens of unwanted rules and regulations. No doubt some discipline is necessary to keep up a daily practice routine. But it will be encouraged only for enriching our life in the here-and-now, not to place undue burdens for the sake of some future enlightenment that we may never find. If there is such a thing as enlightenment, we will find it in gradually increasing measure each day as we continue on our journey of self-directed spiritual practice. We will find it in our career, our family and relationships, and in how we engage in the world in ever more supportive and joyful ways.

Building a Daily Routine (Practice Chart)

How do we go about building a daily routine of spiritual practices? There are a number of places we can start. No doubt, many who are reading here have done so already. It can begin almost anywhere in the *Eight Limbs of Yoga*.

Nowadays, yoga postures (asanas) are very popular. There are millions who have begun on the path of spiritual practices in yoga postures. Maybe this kind of yoga was taken up only for relaxation, for some peace, or for physical fitness. Nevertheless, this is an entry into spiritual practices, as anyone who has been practicing yoga postures for a few years knows.

Maybe spiritual practices began in the form of prayer and worship in our religion, which is an expression of our heartfelt desire to "know God." Raising our desire to a level of devotion to our chosen ideal is a key part of the spiritual path. We all begin there in one way or another. A path without desire is no path at all. A desire for realizing our highest potential does not have to be in a religious context, but it is fine if it is. The methods of yoga do not discriminate. Human spiritual transformation can occur just as well within a religious context as not.

We have all been doing something about our spiritual condition up until now. Just reading this book is an indication that we are considering doing more. But what? In the AYP approach, we aim for efficiency, for optimizing the relationship of causes and effects in spiritual practice. In doing so, we keep the control levers in the hands of the practitioner, where they belong. With the practitioner (you) in control, the practice routine can be built step-by-step, and managed in a way that provides for maximum progress with good comfort and safety. No one else can be driving our car along the highway for us, we have to do it ourselves. It is a long journey we are on, a marathon, not a sprint, and we travel step-by-step.

Basic Routine of Practices

In the AYP approach to practices we begin with deep meditation. So no matter where we may have begun our practices in the past, if we choose to utilize the AYP system, deep meditation will be the suggested starting point. Once we are established in twice-daily deep meditation, the entry into additional practices may follow flexible sequence and timing, according to individual inclinations and experiences. The general <u>sequence of learning</u> (not sequence of doing) looks something like this:

- Deep Meditation
- Spinal Breathing Pranayama
- Asanas (postures)
- Mudras and Bandhas
- Samyama

We do not undertake all this in a week or a few months, and not even in a year, or several years. It takes us months at least to assimilate each of the categories of practice listed. Within each category there are multiple elements of practice which can be implemented over time, so the list is very simplified. But it gives an idea.

Deep meditation and samyama are primarily for cultivating inner silence. Spinal breathing pranayama, asanas, mudras and bandhas are primarily concerned with cultivating the energetic side of our neurobiology, leading the rise of ecstatic conductivity. Together, inner silence and ecstatic conductivity form the two essential building blocks of enlightenment. It is the merging or *marriage* of these two that fulfills the promise of yoga, which is union, expressed as *Oneness* or *Unity* – the actualization of *stillness in action* in everyday living.

The above-mentioned practices comprise our compact twice-daily practice routine. In addition, our normal daily activity constitutes part of practice also, for this is the time we are naturally integrating what we have gained in our *sitting practices*. It is one thing to be cultivating inner silence and ecstatic conductivity during practices, and something else to be stabilizing these qualities as we go about our daily business in life. So keeping an active life is very important.

Besides engaging in daily practices and keeping active, there are additional methods and behaviors we can undertake in our life that will enhance our progress. We will find them rising as *natural tendencies* as we develop more abiding inner silence and natural radiance in our life. They come generally under the *yamas* and *niyamas* in the eight limbs of yoga, and may include:

- A reduction in harmful action
- Increasing honesty in all dealings
- The preservation and cultivation of sexual energy
- A lighter more nutritious diet
- An urge to engage in internal bodily cleansing
- Spiritual study and self-inquiry
- Intense desire for God/Truth
- Greater inclination to serve the needs of others
- More equanimity and contentment in life

This is not to say all of these things will be experienced or undertaken in a systematic way, or that they will happen all at once. It is through our own choices that these things will have a greater tendency to become more a part of our life as our consciousness expands. We will find them creeping into our life naturally as we go about our activities between our daily practice sessions, and our choices will be affected by natural enhancements in our own *seeing*.

Throughout the *AYP writings*, instructions have been provided for these additional behaviors and means. Techniques are provided for the preservation and cultivation of sexual energy (the tools of *tantra*, adaptable to any lifestyle preference – heterosexual, homosexual, solo/masturbation or celibate), diet principles and guidelines (including Ayurveda diet suggestions), shatkarmas (internal cleansing techniques), amaroli (urine therapy), principles and practical guidelines for self-inquiry, the methods of bhakti (use of desire and devotion), and the principles of karma yoga (action in service to our highest ideal).

So there is a wide range of activities that are affected in our life as we undertake daily spiritual practices. Everything, in fact.

What is the return on all this?

Peace and happiness!

And we have to do very little to bring it about. Once we have mustered the desire and a commitment to engage in deep meditation for a few minutes morning and evening, the rest is practically automatic. Once stillness is rising and moving within us, everything will be moving, and we will do as we are inclined to do. All of the resources are available for us to take advantage of as we see fit. That is how self-directed spiritual practice works.

The Practice Chart

In the *Secrets of Wilder* novel, a "plain English" practice chart is provided, covering the main sitting practices of AYP and their relationship to each other in the practice routine. The chart has been updated and expanded, and is included here. In many cases, this updated practice chart provides the original Sanskrit names for practices, and has a number of new features, including additional practices, intentional versus automatic yoga, and other particulars related to balancing a systematic approach with the unique requirements of self-directed spiritual practice. In other words, the AYP approach and the practice chart recognize that one size does not fit all.

The chart can be used for planning and tracking the build-up of our daily practice routine according to our level of experience and inclinations to undertake next steps in a systematic manner.

Let's take a look now.

AYP PRACTICE CHART

Main Practices Sequence* >	Spinal Breathing Pranayama			Energy Cultivation			Deep Meditation			Core Samyama			Energy Cultivation			Cosmic Samyama		
Learning Sequence >	2nd			3rd			1st			4th			5th			6th		
Level** >	B	I	A	B	I	A	B	I	A	B	I	A	B	I	A	B	I	A
Energy Cultivation Practices																		
Mulabandha		I	I						A			A						A
Sambhavi Mudra	I	I	I						A			A						A
Siddhasana		I	I					A	A	A	A							
Uddiyana or Nauli		I	I						A			A						A
Kechari Mudra		I	I						A			A						A
Spinal Bastrika					I	I												
Yoni Mudra				I											I			
Chin Pump					I													
Whole Body Mudra			A			A			A			A			A			A
Practice Times*																		
Standard	5-10 min			2-5 min			10-20 min			5-10 min			2-5 min			5 min		
Aggressive	Over 10 min			Over 5 min			Over 20 min			Over 10 min			Over 5 min			Over 5 min		

Notes:

   * Each cycle of core practices is preceded by asanas (postures), and followed by rest.

  ** Practitioner Level: **B** = Basic, **I** = Intermediate, **A** = Advanced

*** Practice times are twice per day. Structured retreats may include more practice cycles per day.

"I" designates an <u>Intentional Practice</u>

"A" designates an <u>Automatic Practice</u>

The chart is not as complicated as may appear at first glance. Across the top row headings, the main practices are shown, in the order they are performed in each session, going from left to right. In the second row across the top the suggested order of learning the practices is shown, deep meditation first, spinal breathing pranayama second, and so on…

Down the left side of the chart, the various energy-related practices are shown. Near the bottom you will see *Yoni Mudra* and *Chin Pump* in bold. Both of these are multi-faceted practices and can contain most of the energy-related practices listed above them, depending upon the degree to which they are applied.

Whole Body Mudra, also shown in bold at the bottom of the left side column, is not as much a practice as an effect of practices, It has been included because it is an important automatic yoga that arises as our overall practice routine advances, and ecstatic conductivity arises in the neurobiology as a self-sustaining phenomenon.

The grid in the center of the chart shows a *basic*, *intermediate* and *advanced* stage for each of the main practice categories, and indicates which energy-related practices may be occurring as the practitioner becomes more advanced over time. Practices marked in the grid may be designated with an "*I*" representing an intentional practice, or with an "*A*" representing an automatic practice. *Intentional practices* are those we choose to do according to the procedure provided to us in the AYP instructional writings. *Automatic practices* are those that may be experienced naturally during the course of our practice routine, or at other times during the day. Intentional practices are easily favored over automatic practices for reasons that are explained in the self-pacing discussion in the next section of this chapter.

Across the bottom of the chart, typical practice times are shown for both *standard* and *aggressive* approaches to practices. Practice times in the aggressive category may lead to excessive purification and opening in the nervous system, with the corresponding discomforts. Excesses may even be encountered in the standard practice time ranges by those who are sensitive to practices. It always boils down to individual experience and the pacing of practices for maximum progress with comfort. The time ranges shown on the chart are suggestions only and may be adjusted to suit individual capacity and need.

The practice chart is not intended to represent anything absolute about our practice routine. It is a visual tool to aid us in building a practice routine that will work best for us.

Finding Detailed Instructions for the Practices

Obviously, it is not possible to include detailed instructions for all the practices pointed to in this short book. Here we are looking at the key elements of effective practice and suggesting how they can be structured into an effective integrated routine for the long term. Instructions for doing the individual practices are provided throughout the *AYP writings*, which serious practitioners will want to study in their entirety.

Lessons providing detailed instructions for the practices on the chart can be found in the *AYP Easy Lessons for Ecstatic Living* textbook by looking them up in the *Topic Index* in the last section of the book, or in the *Topic Index* provided on the main AYP website.

The *AYP Enlightenment Series* books provide clear and concise instructions for the core practices of AYP, as indicated by the book titles and content descriptions found on the *Books Page* of the AYP website.

Also, the *Secrets of Wilder* novel is a story set in modern times covering the discovery and application of the practices, providing readers the opportunity to vicariously travel the path of practices and human spiritual transformation.

For further reading and support on all of the practices, see the last page of this book.

Building Our Routine – Sequence and Timing

We have provided a structure here, and the particulars of many powerful practices throughout the *AYP writings*. We have also provided strong reasons for implementing an integration of daily practices (the whole is greater than the sum of the parts), and suggested a step-by-step sequence for accomplishing that. Yet, with all that information, it still boils down to each of us finding our own best application of daily practices that is compatible with our inclinations and lifestyle. This is why we call it *self-directed spiritual practice*. Who can know better what will work best for us? We will find out as we take each step in applying all that we have learned, and we will make the necessary adjustments along the way.

If we follow the AYP approach, there will be many choices for us to make. If we are combining the AYP approach with practices we have been doing, or plan to do in the future, we will be engaged in a research project of much greater complexity with many more choices. Obviously, the latter is not for beginners, or even intermediate practitioners.

Let's say we are starting today pretty much from scratch. We have had some bhakti (spiritual desire) brewing for some time and have begun daily deep meditation.

What next?

As we look at the practice chart, we may be tempted to jump into spinal breathing pranayama right away, and maybe throw in some energy cultivation practices for good measure.

Not a very good idea.

The next step after beginning deep meditation is stabilizing our twice-daily routine before taking on any additional practices. This is the guideline for undertaking any new practice – stabilize it for a period of time.

How long?

The time needed to stabilize any given practice will vary according to the unique pattern of purification and opening that will be occurring in each person. So we have to gauge it for ourselves. We will know how we are doing by how we feel during our daily activity. Results in daily living are the measure of our practice, not what we might experience during practices. Experiences in practices can be anything, and are nearly always symptoms of purification and opening. This may come as a shock to those who have engaged in yoga mainly for the flashy experiences. Practices can produce plenty of these, and we will be wise to regard them as *scenery* along the road to enlightenment. If we become overly attached to experiences, we could fall off our practices, the source of our progress.

Experiences do not produce enlightenment. Practices do.

It is a common pitfall, like taking on too many practices at once. In time, we develop a maturity in considering all of our possibilities, and how to best proceed in unfolding them.

Step-by-step... We cannot do it all in the first day, month or year. If we try for that, we will stumble for sure. That's okay, as long as we know how to make the necessary adjustments and carry on. We will discuss this in more detail in the next section on self-pacing.

So, let's suppose we have been doing deep meditation like clockwork for a few months and things are going well. We have made it through our clunky beginning stage with the *I AM* mantra, practice is smoothing out, and we are noticing some inner silence in our daily activity. Not bad.

What now?

This is a time when we can consider taking on spinal breathing pranayama, which will enliven our deep meditation, adding a dynamic quality to the stillness we are cultivating deep within. For those who may not be inclined to take on spinal breathing, an alternative approach (not shown on the practice chart) would be adding core samyama instead of spinal breathing or other energy cultivation practices. It all depends on our individual nature and tendency.

For those who have taken on deep meditation, spinal breathing pranayama and additional practices, and have finally come to spinal bastrika, then this practice can be done either after spinal breathing (as shown on the practice chart), or before spinal breathing, which is an alternative place for it to be located in the overall practice routine. In either place it will be equally effective, and it is a matter of personal choice.

The AYP practices are not cast in stone. We are cultivating inner silence and ecstatic conductivity. Deep meditation and spinal breathing pranayama will do this. Deep meditation and samyama will do it also, assuming our nervous system is sufficiently conditioned to support ecstatic conductivity. The most reliable approach for cultivating inner silence and ecstatic conductivity is building a balanced blend of mental, breathing, and physical techniques. As discussed earlier, there are additional things we can develop outside sitting practices – tantra, self-inquiry, service, etc.

While we would all like an exact blueprint for building our practice routine, it will depend a lot on our own tendencies. What we have offered here is a tentative blueprint that can work for a large cross-section of serious seekers. It is flexible, and can be adapted and adjusted in many ways to suit individual patterns of purification and opening.

It should be pointed out that there are limits to how flexible the AYP (or any system) can be. If one begins deep meditation, and then goes off into adding on multiple practices from multiple systems, expecting to find a shortcut to enlightenment, there will be a greatly reduced chance of sustaining steady and stable progress. In fact, such a random approach can lead to much discomfort and confusion, and much less progress. So, while the AYP system is flexible, it is not a blank check for doing anything and everything.

Likewise, if the AYP approach is applied with limited flexibility, disregarding the effects of practices in daily activity, there can be difficulties with that. By *flexibility*, we mean a good application of common sense in taking on practices in a progressive and comfortable fashion.

Self-Pacing

With a twice-daily routine of practices, we place ourselves on a fast track to enlightenment. It is potentially so fast that it is essential we develop skill in regulating the practices we are doing each day, measuring duration in time or repetitions, depending on the practice. We adjust practice duration as necessary to maintain smooth and steady progress without incurring excessive discomfort due to too many obstructions being released in our nervous system.

This regulation of practices is called *self-pacing*, and it too is a practice – one of the most important in the entire AYP arsenal. For, without good self-pacing, we are not likely to get very far on the road to enlightenment.

Practical Application of Self-Pacing

A key aspect of practices is the prudent handling of experiences, whether they are mundane, dramatic, or extreme. This is a path of enjoyment, and we are entitled to enjoy the *scenery* we encounter on our journey to enlightenment. However, the scenery is not what will advance us on our path. It is our practices that will move us ahead. So, after an admiring look at the passing scenery, no matter how beautiful or attention-grabbing it may be, we easily go back to the practice we are doing. If spiritual experiences come while we are in our daily activities, as they certainly shall, we can then continue to enjoy the experiences, or go back to whatever it is we are doing.

If experiences become extreme or uncomfortable, either during practice, or afterward in our daily activity, the advice is to scale back our practice in order to bring things back in balance. For example, if we have gotten carried away with our deep meditation practice and are meditating for too long in our twice-daily routine, it is possible that we will experience headache or irritability during our daily activity.

It can also happen if we are getting up too quickly after practices, without an adequate rest period at the end. There is a direct cause and effect between our practices and our experiences in daily life. If we are finding discomfort, then it is time to reduce practices sufficiently and make sure we are taking adequate rest at the end to restore balance. If we have been practicing a normal amount and find some imbalance, then the scaling back can be temporary. As our adverse symptoms subside, then we can creep back to our normal level of practice. However, if we have been overdoing to the extreme, and suffering the consequences, then we should adjust our practice times to levels that are reasonable, so we can continue to live a normal life, while naturally integrating the benefits of our practices into our everyday activities. This will yield the best long term results for us.

We always have a choice. Spiritual life is not something that must be hijacking us from ordinary life. If it is, we have probably been engaged in excess, either recently or at some time in the past, and establishing a stable routine of practices can correct this. Spiritual life is something that can be cultivated to bring fulfillment to our activities in everyday life, whatever they may be. We are free to live our rising spiritual experiences in a way that is compatible with our needs. It is our life, our journey, and our enlightenment. We have no one to become but our *Self*.

Automatic Yoga – Physical Movements

The methods of yoga have been derived over the centuries from the natural capabilities for spiritual unfoldment contained within every human nervous system. Yoga does not determine these inherent capabilities. It optimizes the application of them.

As we embark on a path of daily practice, it will not be unusual for us to experience various expressions of our inner capabilities for purification and opening. We are stimulating the spiritual neurobiology, so it is natural for there to be some response. Ultimately, the response will be wide-ranging, because the connectivity of yoga exists between every organ, nerve and cell in our body. With systematic stimulation in daily practices, the connections will awaken and there will be movement.

The movement may come in the form of rising interest in all things spiritual – a desire to study and do more to enhance our progress on our spiritual path. It can also come in the form of an inner ecstatic energy flow, or other energy symptoms.

The movement can also be quite literal at times, in the form of physical movements and postures that may occur automatically during our regular routine of practices, and sometimes outside practices. These physical manifestations of yoga connectivity within us are referred to as *automatic yoga*.

Some symptoms of automatic yoga may include rapid breathing (bastrika) or a slowdown or stoppage of breath (kumbhaka), the head going forward, back, or around (forms of jalandhara), the torso of the body going forward and down during sitting practices (yoga mudra), other mudras or bandhas, vibrations of the body, rapid movement of the legs and/or arms, vocalizations of various kinds, and many other things. Or there may be nothing at all. Just gradually more inner silence, energy and happiness in daily living.

Those who have experiences of automatic yoga are not necessarily more advanced or gifted than those who do not. Automatic yoga is part of the process of inner purification and opening occurring as a result of yoga practices, and nothing more than that. For some it will be more pronounced than for others. Those who are not shaking all over the place will be purifying and opening within in ways that are appropriate for the unique matrix of obstructions that is present in the their nervous system. Some are purified through study, some are purified through increasing devotion or other sensations that express the inner divine, and some are purified through physical movements. Regardless of the symptoms that may be occurring, <u>all are purified and opened through the systematic application of daily yoga practices.</u>

If physical movements or other symptoms are occurring within our practices, or outside them, what are we supposed to do? In practices, it is the same as any thought, vision or sensation that may occur. When we notice our attention has drifted off the practice we are doing, we just easily come back to the practice. If we are doing deep meditation, we easily come back to the mantra. If we are doing spinal breathing pranayama, we just easily come back to tracing the breath between root and brow. If we are engaged in asanas, we just easily favor the posture we are doing.

If automatic yoga becomes overwhelming, we can ease off our practice for a few minutes and let our attention easily be with the sensations we are experiencing. This will usually settle the energy down. Then we can go back to our practice. If physical symptoms continue to be intense, we can lay down and rest for a while.

All purification passes, and all symptoms of energy movements will settle down in time, as our nervous system gradually becomes a purer conductor of the vast inner energies we are awakening with yoga practices. While automatic yoga during normal daily activity is less common, it can happen sometimes. In that case it is the same as any other spiritual experiences we may have. We can allow the experiences while observing them without excessive participation or judgment, or we can just go on with our daily activities. In time all such symptoms will smooth out and become synonymous with the divine flow of our life. We always have the choice. Automatic yoga can only dominate if we will it to.

In some systems of practice there are certain times when automatic yoga in the form of physical movements may be permitted to occur as part of the practice. In the AYP system of practices, this would be during samyama, during the *lightness sutra*, and to lesser degrees during other sitting practices, where we do not fight against swaying and other occasional spontaneous movements that might occur during the normal course of our practices. This does not mean we depart from our practice and focus our full attention on the automatic yoga. This can be counterproductive, leading to overdoing, particularly with changes in breathing or suspensions of breath.

It is good to keep in mind that automatic yoga is not going to be cognizant of our limit for accommodating purification and opening in a given period of time. Rather, automatic yoga is an impulse to have it all right now. This is not possible without a high probability of undergoing extreme discomfort, and then not being able to continue. In yoga it is always best to let common sense have the last say, particularly when the impulses that will lead us into excess are stirring. So we always favor our structured routine of practices, come what may, and then we will be assured of good progress with the least amount of disruption. This is how our process of inner purification and opening will continue to move forward. We always easily favor the practice over the experience.

If there are few a surges, bends or jerks occurring along the way, this will be normal, as will be the lack of them. It is all part of our natural unfoldment.

The Hazards of Forcing Practices

In life, we have all had the urge to "go for it" at one time or other, to push hard to reach our objective. In many fields of human endeavor, it is considered a virtue to follow this impulse – the proverbial race for the finish line in whatever we are doing. It is the stuff that heroes are made of.

But not in yoga, where the hero is the one who is able to let go of acts of desperation in practices and allow the natural process of purification and opening to occur with the least amount of disruption.

Forcing yoga practices leads to excess in symptoms of purification and the associated discomforts. If forcing has been extreme, particularly when jumping too far ahead in undertaking advanced practices, then the discomfort can be extensive, to the point where practices must stop.

Symptoms of overdoing in practices are due to excessive purification occurring in the nervous system related to premature awakening of *kundalini*. The symptoms can be mental, emotional, physical, or any combination of these. Kundalini, the source of great ecstasy within us, can also bring great discomfort, if approached carelessly. The consideration of kundalini, its symptoms of excess, and associated remedies, is a broad and complex subject that is fully covered in the *AYP writings*. If yoga practices are applied in a logical sequence with prudent self-pacing, the excesses and suffering associated with a premature kundalini awakening can be largely avoided.

Assistance for handling excesses when they do occur is available in the *AYP Support Forums*. Many of the cases addressed there result from excesses developed in other systems of spiritual practice, where optimal integration of practices and self-pacing are little understood or applied. For those who have developed skill in using the AYP approach, such extremes have been rare.

When symptoms of inner energy imbalance become excessive, then special measures are necessary to recover before the spiritual journey can continue. In this way, forcing our practices can lead to a significant slowdown in our spiritual progress, not to mention the unnecessary discomfort. While we are recovering from overdoing, the clock will continue to run.

Sometimes, forcing and overdoing in practices will not produce immediate uncomfortable symptoms, leading instead to a <u>delayed reaction</u> that can be quite severe. This is especially true with pranayama and breath suspension (kumbhaka) methods. In fact, there can be pleasurable symptoms when first overdoing, inspiring the practitioner to take the overdoing to a further extreme. And then, wham!

So it is very important for us to establish a stable routine of practices that we can sustain over the long term, adding on in small steps from time to time when we are sure that we are ready. This measured approach is the fastest and most reliable way to cultivate spiritual progress.

If we are driving too fast in our car along a winding mountain road and fly off a cliff, we will be hard-pressed to reach our destination in a timely manner. On the other hand, if we are prudent and drive our car skillfully at a safe speed, we will be sure to reach our destination on schedule.

Grounding for Stability

If we have overdone it a bit in practices, we will know to scale back on our practice times until the imbalance of our inner energies has been resolved. An important part of this has to do with our daily activity.

Even with a good stable routine of sitting practices, our daily activity is very important. The inner silence we cultivate in deep meditation and the inner energy awakening we stimulate with spinal breathing pranayama and other practices must be stabilized in regular daily activity. This is very important so we can integrate these inner spiritual qualities in our everyday life. It is natural for inner silence and the inner energies to seek an outer expression in the world. Whatever we are doing during the day between our practices will become that path. So it is essential to maintain an active life according to our own inclinations. Then our inner qualities will become increasingly stable in all that we do, bringing a peacefulness, creativity and energy to all aspects of our daily activity.

So grounding is fundamental to all spiritual practice, though we may not call it that as we going about our normal activities.

When there is an excess of inner energy due to overdoing in our yoga practices, or for other reasons, it is wise to scale back on practices temporarily, and ramp up our grounding activities. This can mean regular physical exercise, more engagement in social activity, chores around the house, digging in the garden, doing a daily Tai Chi routine, eating a heavier diet, whatever it takes to ground ourselves. During such times, it will also be wise to scale back on spiritual study and devotional activities, which can also over-stimulate our inner energies.

All of these will be temporary measures, until we find our balance in daily living again. As we do, we can gradually restore our practices and adjust our daily activities according to what is necessary to maintain steady long term progress with comfort and safety.

Self-Pacing and Physical Practices

What we are talking about here is the application of good common sense. Self-pacing applies in many aspects of our life. The successful application of yoga practices is no different than anything else. If we overdo, we pay the price.

Not surprisingly, self-pacing in yoga practices applies across the board, whether we are talking about deep meditation, breathing methods or anything else, including the level of our devotion (bhakti), the intensity of our spiritual studies, our dietary preferences, or measures we might take to purify our body by physical means (shatkarmas). Wherever we happen to be working on the tree of yoga, the principles of self-pacing apply.

In modern times, many are coming to yoga through training in physical postures (asanas). When considering asanas, or related physical practices like mudras and bandhas, if there is some stiffness, injury, or discomfort, then we just go to our natural limit and test it a little. Never to the point of pain or strain. Just to the point of the limit of movement, and then be there for the time of our posture. This may be nowhere near the full posture, which is perfectly fine. We do what we can comfortably in the direction of the posture without strain, knowing we will be doing gradually more in subsequent sessions. If any degree of stretch becomes uncomfortable, we back off to a comfortable level. Or, if it can go a little further without strain, then we let it. This is what we have talked about many times as we have gone through the many AYP practices.

It is the same with all yoga practices – physical, mental, breathing, etc. All practices produce purification and opening in our nervous system, and we are obliged to accommodate whatever is happening on our journey to enlightenment. It is the principle of self-pacing. It is the fine art of progressing in yoga – never forcing, always using gentle persuasion. With this approach, the body, nervous system, heart and mind move slowly but surely to more flexibility, purification, and greater experiences of inner peace and bliss.

There is the old saying, "By the yard, life is hard. By the inch, it's a cinch."

It is easy to become advanced in yoga if we know how to handle self-pacing.

Keeping up Practices with a Busy Schedule

Whatever system of spiritual practices we are following, chances are that we have heard, or figured out on our own, that daily practice is the key to success. The journey of human spiritual transformation takes time, and the inner changes that lead to our enlightenment require daily cultivation. Daily spiritual practices are also needed when we already have spiritual momentum, meaning, we have some degree of dynamic inner opening occurring either through previous practices, or a *spontaneous awakening*. If we rely only on the energies that are moving in us spontaneously, then we can be prone to imbalances that will make our journey homeward toward unending ecstatic bliss and divine love considerably less comfortable, and potentially longer than necessary.

So, no matter what our approach or level of attainment is, reaching our destination in a reliable fashion depends on having daily spiritual practices firmly in place. This has been a central theme throughout the *AYP writings*, beginning with the first instructions on deep meditation, and with many reminders since then.

Honoring the Habit of Twice-Daily Practice

In the original instructions on deep meditation and spinal breathing pranayama, suggestions are provided on how to fit these practices into a busy schedule. Wherever we may be, we can close our eyes and meditate – in trains, airplanes, waiting rooms, just about anywhere. The same is true for spinal breathing pranayama. If we are willing to be flexible and compromise on our practices from time to time, we can keep up the habit under the most adverse circumstances. There is great value in this, for it assures us of a continuation of practices over the long term, which is the key to our enlightenment.

We do not live in an ideal world. Even with the best plans for regular practice in our meditation room, it can all go out the window with a family emergency or other intervening events. Does this mean our daily practices have to go out the window too? Not if we have a strategy. There are ways to keep our practices going, no matter what is happening.

As our routine of practices becomes more sophisticated, involving more practices, keeping it all going in a busy schedule presents both challenges and opportunities. With so many pieces to work with in an advanced routine, we can be pretty creative in compressing our practices when time is short. Where there is the will, there is a way!

Let's talk about the basics of establishing and keeping a habit of doing daily spiritual practices. One of the easiest ways to do it is make a rule for ourselves that we will do our routine before we eat breakfast and dinner – twice each day like that. If the time of one or both of those meals isn't stable, then we can tag it to be done upon awakening in the morning, and as soon as we arrive home in the evening. If we are traveling, it gets a bit more complicated, but practices can be done to some degree under just about any circumstance, as long as we honor our habit.

Keeping the habit is not about always doing a full routine. It does not have to be "all or nothing." The habit is an urge we build into ourselves to do something about spiritual practice at the appointed time that comes twice-daily. Having the habit is having the *urge to practice*. This cultivated urge is the seed of all daily practice. It is like getting hungry at meal times. It just happens, and we want to eat. If we have the urge for spiritual practices cultivated like that, then we will do them. Most days we will be doing our whole routine. On other days, we may be doing less. But we will always be doing something every session. This "always doing something every session" is very important.

To illustrate what we mean by *honoring the habit*, let's suppose we are hurrying down a busy street. We are on our way to a business dinner appointment that will tie us up until bedtime. We are walking quickly, weaving our way through the people we are passing on the sidewalk. The restaurant is just around the corner now. Almost there.

But wait! We see a bench, an empty bus stop bench on the sidewalk in the middle of all the people hurrying this way and that way. We have that urge built into us to do practices. It is time. So what do we do? We stop and sit on that bench for a few minutes and meditate. It might be only for two minutes. But why not? Who will miss us for those two minutes? And we have kept our habit to sit. It is amazing how doing something small like that can renew us for an entire evening – centering for just a few minutes, picking up the mantra just a few times. The nervous system says, "Thank you!" And we are calmer for the rest of the evening.

But it is not just about centering for a few minutes. It is also about keeping our habit of twice-daily practices. If we are in a crazy schedule for days or weeks like that, and can just sit for a few minutes before breakfast and dinner, then when we recover control of our schedule we won't be struggling to find our practice routine again. The habit will be there, and then we can indulge it with our full routine, which we know will fill us to overflowing with inner silence and divine ecstasy.

So that is the first thing – keeping the habit, even if it for two minutes on a bus stop bench. It does not matter where it is, or what is going on. We can keep the habit if we are committed. Then it will keep us committed, because it becomes a hunger that comes on its own at the appointed time. Then we will not have to struggle to restore our commitment to yoga once we are free to do twice-daily full routines of practice again. It is more likely that we will be faced with compromises in our practice time that are not usually as extreme as having to take a few minutes on a bus stop bench. Let's talk about those.

Optimizing the Practice Time We Have

If we are doing spinal breathing pranayama and deep meditation, followed by a few minutes of rest while coming out, it is not difficult to tailor our practice to a time limitation. Say we are doing 10 minutes of spinal breathing, 20 minutes of meditation, and 5 minutes of rest. That is a 35 minute routine. Then one day we may find ourselves with only 15 minutes to work with. We can just do 10 minutes of meditation, rest for a few minutes and get up. We can also put a few minutes of spinal breathing in front. If we know we will be short on time, we can start with some light spinal breathing while walking to our meditation seat. If we have to choose between spinal breathing and meditation, we always choose meditation. One thing we do not do is combine spinal breathing and deep meditation at the same time. This will reduce the effectiveness of both practices, deep meditation especially.

Let's suppose we have progressed to the point where we are doing a "full plate" of practices – everything shown on the practice chart, to a moderate degree. So let's lay it out. It is a typical routine. If you are doing more or less of any of the practices, then you can make the necessary adjustments in translating the suggestions on what to do when the schedule crunch hits you. The idea is to develop some strategies that will enable us to keep our routine together when time is short. Think about it in advance: "What will I do if my practice time is cut in half?" There is no absolute right or wrong answer. Beyond a few basics, keeping practices going when time is short is an art. So here is our "full plate" routine:

- Asanas – 10 min
- Spinal breathing – 10 min
- Chin pump – 2-3 min
- Spinal bastrika – 2-3 min
- Meditation – 20 min
- Samyama (core) – 10 min
- Yoni mudra – 2-3 minutes
- Cosmic Samyama – 5 minutes (lying down)
- Rest – 5 min or more (lying down)

That is a little over an hour. There is nothing sacred about the times in this routine. Maybe you are doing five minutes of spinal breathing, and no samyama. Or maybe no asanas. Or no chin pump. Maybe no cosmic samyama. Whatever the combination is, it is up to you. Just make sure you are not skipping meditation or rest. Those two (cultivation of inner silence, plus a stable transition to daily activity) are the foundation of all spiritual progress. Spinal breathing is right behind meditation and rest in importance. So, spinal breathing, meditation, and ending rest by themselves constitute a powerful routine of practices. All the rest of the practices are for enhancing and building on the effects of these. This *pecking order* is what we use as a guideline when it is necessary for us to begin compressing our practice routine into a tighter schedule.

So, let's say we have this wonderful one-hour-plus practice routine, and all of a sudden, due to circumstances beyond our control, we find ourselves with only thirty minutes to do our afternoon routine. Without a plan, the inclination might be to just bag it for the afternoon and try again tomorrow. All or nothing, you know. That is not a good strategy. Not only will we lose the benefit of a skillfully compressed routine, but we will also dilute our habit to practice twice-daily. The urge to practice needs twice-daily reinforcement. Just remember the bus stop bench. If a few minutes on a bench was good enough to keep the habit going, isn't thirty minutes in a relatively quiet room a luxury? It really is. So here are some suggestions on what we can do.

First, we hang on to meditation. That is always the first priority. But we'd like to do some of the other practices too, so let's trim the meditation to 15 minutes in this 30 minute plan. We know we need up to five minutes of rest at the end for a smooth transition back into activity, so that is 20 minutes, leaving us with 10 minutes to work with. Next is spinal breathing. We can do five minutes of spinal breathing in front of meditation and then use the remaining five minutes for other things. Which practice should the last five minutes be for?

At this point, it depends on our preference. If we love our samyama, then we can go for five minutes of that and leave asanas, chin pump and yoni mudra for tomorrow.

Additionally, in less than one minute before we sit for practices, we can do a standing *abbreviated asana routine* that includes bending back, twisting left and right, and bending forward and touching toes. A little uddiyana and/or nauli can be done then also. All of the elements of an asana routine can be touched on in this way in about a minute. It is far from optimal, but it is something in the asanas department we can do before we sit.

So, in this way, we can do a pretty good routine in 30 minutes if we are faced with a time limit like that. It can be done in less time too. Of course, then we are dropping more practices off. But we can always do something, even if it is sitting on a bus stop bench for a few minutes, picking up the mantra and dipping into pure bliss consciousness.

Is should be mentioned that we don't have to give up the energy-related practices that are done in parallel (at the same time) while we are sitting in spinal breathing and deep meditation, because they do not take any extra time. These may include siddhasana, mulabandha, sambhavi mudra and kechari mudra. To the extent we are practicing these, they can always be incorporated with our core sitting practices in every session, no matter how short the time is. Indeed, they will be found creeping into our everyday activity as ecstatic conductivity is coming up in our nervous system. By then, mudras and bandhas have become part of our normal neurobiological functioning, coming up automatically as ecstatic micro-movements deep within us in a coordinated way, and we will never lose them. This is what we mean by *whole body mudra*.

Of course, we have to be mindful about practices we are doing in public view. Doing chin pump in a busy airport waiting room could be rather conspicuous. But most of our practices can be done discreetly. That certainly applies to light spinal breathing, meditation, samyama, mulabandha, and kechari. Sambhavi is not noticeable if done with eyes closed, which is recommended anyway. The abbreviated standing asana routine can be done without much fanfare. It is only stretching, which everyone will understand. Even siddhasana can be done discreetly in a public place if one shoe is removed and our heel is slipped up under our perineum. Sometimes where we happen to be will determine what practices we will do. As the old saying goes: "Discretion is the better part of valor."

There are many ways to piece together practices if we are faced with a short schedule, or less than ideal location. After spinal breathing, meditation, and ending rest are taken care of, it is up to our personal preferences. Give it some thought. When the need arises, we can find interesting and creative ways to keep our practices going. With bhakti, we will find a way.

In this busy world, we will all be faced with the challenge of having limited time for our practices. As we continue with yoga, our spiritual desire (bhakti) will become stronger, and we will find ways to keep the necessary time available. Even so, there will be things that come up occasionally that will limit our time, so it is wise to develop an attitude of flexibility and a willingness to compromise when necessary to make sure that we are always honoring our habit to practice twice each day. If we do that, there won't be much in this world that can keep us from reaching our divine destination.

Group Practice and Retreats

Spiritual enthusiasm (bhakti) is wonderful, and we can use it to enhance our practices for sure. However, as discussed earlier in this chapter, it can be hazardous to suddenly lengthen our sessions or add on additional practices. This is pressing the envelope of what our nervous system can accommodate in a given time period. Any change should be done gradually, with each step stabilized and sustained as part of our regular routine over weeks and months before making additional changes. The key to success in yoga practices is long term consistency and stability in our routine, with gradual adjustments occurring from time to time.

For those who would like to increase inspiration and knowledge, as well as safely enhance spiritual progress beyond daily practices at home, structured group meditations and retreats can be very helpful.

Group Meditations

Group meditations are a good thing. Any gathering that is for the purpose of studying and encouraging paths of spiritual unfoldment can be good. If there can be some communications with others of like interest on a regular basis, there can be significant benefits, particularly in inspiring us to press forward with our daily practices. Likewise, we can inspire others to practice as well.

The forming of meditation groups is encouraged, meeting once per week or so. Such meetings can begin with a group meditation of ten minutes at the beginning and then open discussion on practice and experiences with some refreshments being served, as desired. Group meditations have their own quality. They can be deep and pervasive as multiple quieting minds mingle and reinforce each other. It is a noticeable effect, and radiates outward to the surroundings. Group meditations are good for individual meditators, and uplifting for the world.

At times we may find ourselves at meditation meetings involving practices other than deep meditation. Some people go for "guided meditations." This style of group meditation is not compatible with using the mantra in deep meditation, because our practice is for going inward quickly and efficiently. As deep meditation with mantra becomes habit, we will be gone within as soon as we close our eyes. A talking meditation guide will then be counter-productive. The same goes for meditations using music, chanting, drumming, etc. These all have their purpose and benefits, but are not compatible with taking the mantra inward quickly to pure bliss consciousness. This is not to say we shouldn't participate in guided meditations, chanting, or whatever. But it will be a distinctly different procedure from our daily meditation with mantra, or a deep meditation group.

If a deep meditation group is not available in your area, then start one. There is assistance available for this in the *AYP Support Forums* at the link provided on the last page of this book.

Jesus said, "For where two or three are gathered in my name, there I am in the midst of them."

This quote is not given from a sectarian point of view. It describes a well-known principle. When people gather for a spiritual purpose, consciousness is stimulated and rises. This rising can be experienced as deepening inner silence and pervading pure bliss consciousness. This experience occurs in every gathering for a high spiritual ideal, in every gathering for truth. The group experience of pervading inner silence is maximized during group meditations.

Group meditations are not a substitute for our regular twice-daily meditations. Our individual practice is our primary practice, and it should always be. This keeps our spiritual destiny in our hands, regardless of other circumstances. Group meditations can be a wonderful boost, but they will come and go in our life as circumstances change around us. Don't rely on them as core practice. Think of them as bonuses.

Life is always changing on the outside. Let's be sure that our daily practice is ingrained as an inside aspect of our life, not subject to being waylaid by outer events. We have talked about the various strategies for sustaining daily meditation practice in non-routine situations, with a busy schedule, and so on. Keeping our regularity in practice is very important as we travel along the road of life. Whatever we ultimately choose our daily practice to be, this should be sacred. It is our primary pathway inward. We can count on it, because we are committed to doing it every day without fail. Everything else is passing scenery, inspiring at times, and not so inspiring at other times. Lean toward the inspiring, let it light the fire of desire for progress, and let daily practices continue to do the work of ongoing inner purification and opening. A daily routine is the key. It is the surest path to enlightenment.

Group Samyama

Samyama is a systematic practice of releasing specific words or phrases (*sutras*) in stillness, which leads to positive influences flowing outward from within our stillness. This accelerates our inner purification and opening, and also can produce purifying effects in our environment, both nearby and at great distances. We call this influence from samyama practice *stillness in action*. Traditionally in yoga, these external effects are called *siddhis*.

Group samyama can be performed where there is a common cause that several or many deep meditation practitioners may wish to join together on. For example, if a friend is ill, their name can be used in group samyama practice, and beneficial healing energy will automatically be coming their way. Group samyama can also be performed with our core samyama practice right after a group meditation, if the practitioners present are using samyama during their regular daily routine at home.

Group practice of samyama can also be performed by many practitioners around the world by coordinating the time of practice over the internet. This is, in fact, being done in the *AYP Support Forums*, where many across the globe are engaging in group meditations and samyama sessions every week. All are welcome to join in these sessions to aid those in need, and to help uplift the whole of humanity.

Retreats

By *retreat*, we mean stepping away from our normal daily routine of activities and undertaking a specific schedule designed for enhancing our spiritual progress in an accelerated way. This can be done in solo mode or with a group. For those who are not experienced in retreats, joining a group retreat is preferred, where everything will be taken care of and we can follow the pre-determined schedule for maximum benefit.

On a retreat, there is the possibility to systematically increase the number of meditations we do in a day. This can be to repeat our entire routine of practices a second time in the morning – adding one routine of practice for one or two days on a weekend or holiday, or on an ongoing basis if on an extended retreat. This adds a large degree of purification, and deep momentum in spiritual progress. Being free of responsibilities is very important to do this, or it can lead to discomfort and unpleasant experiences because so much is being released from inside. If we do three routines in a day it is essential to have some light activity in-between the morning and evening sessions, such as non-strenuous walking and gentle (social) *satsang*. This light activity helps balance the process of release of obstructions from the nervous system.

For two morning routines, the basic sequence of practices is asanas, pranayama, deep meditation, samyama (if doing it), rest (at least 10 minutes lying down)... and then start over. In the evening only one routine should be done. This is three full routines of practice in a day.

Three routines per day is an ambitious schedule, especially with a group. Keep in mind that group practice brings extra purifying effects in and of itself, even with our normal routine of doing two practice sessions per day. First time group retreats, where both the leaders and participants are new to retreats with the AYP practices, are best undertaken with two practice routines per day. If all goes well, a more ambitious schedule can be considered for subsequent retreats.

Do not be surprised if a lot of purification and opening occurs during a retreat. While advanced yoga practices are very simple, they are very powerful – especially when performed in groups. If releases become too much, then back off practices to a more stable routine immediately, and advise the retreat leaders of any difficulties. Always keep self-pacing in mind.

A typical daily sequence of events for an AYP retreat would encompass the following:

- Rise (hygiene and light snack as needed)
- Morning Practices
- Study or Meeting Activity
- Lunch
- Light Physical Activity (walking)
- Study or Meeting Activity
- Rest
- Evening Practices
- Dinner
- Study or Meeting Activity
- Bed

The specific timing for each of these activities is provided by the retreat leaders. Sticking to a predetermined schedule is the most important rule of a retreat, and it should be adhered to as closely as possible. It is recommended not to add new practices or extensions in time of current practices while on retreat, except as may be instructed by the retreat leaders.

The beneficial effects of a retreat can be noticed for weeks or months after the retreat is over. It is like adding a longer cycle of purification and opening underneath our normal daily cycle. A retreat adds a large wave of inner silence underneath us. If we attend weekend or week-long retreats two or more times per year, it can add a significant boost to our overall spiritual progress over the long term.

More information on leading and participating in retreats can be found in the *AYP Support Forums*.

Our Role as Teachers and Researchers

We stand at a critical juncture in the history of human spiritual development. We are moving from a very long time of superstition and second-hand knowledge, to a time of direct knowledge based on first hand experience with practices. More importantly, we are taking responsibility for our own spiritual unfoldment through a scientific approach to practices, where causes and effects can be observed and optimized for best effects in each of us individually, and in all of us collectively. It is a major change from how things have been done in the past, leading to a huge increase in the availability and effectiveness of practices for all time to come.

There have been those who have said that human beings are not capable of managing their own spiritual unfoldment, and that this responsibility must be delegated to *those who know*, with no room for choices or adjustments by the practitioner. The results of this approach have been inefficient, and history speaks for itself in this regard. It is time for change.

Responsibility

The journey of purification and opening requires prudent regulation of practices. Only the practitioner can do that. So it is about responsibility. The level of responsibility shown by those who have taken up the AYP open source system of practices has been impressive.

There have been perennial predictions that open knowledge of spiritual practices would lead to disastrous results. It is not true, at least not here and now. Self-pacing is a concept and a practice that is easy to understand and apply. The "learning to drive the fast car" analogy is one we can all relate to, where self-regulation of our speed is necessary under different driving conditions for us to maintain good progress with safety on our journey. It is the same with applying powerful spiritual practices.

The tendency toward desperation and overdoing in practices is driven more by the lack of effective practices than by the open availability of them. What is withheld we tend become desperate for, and we often overcompensate with the practices we do have.

What is freely available we must develop the skill to use responsibly, and we will. It is that simple.

So, there is much to be thankful for as we continue to move forward responsibly with our practices, going step-by-step. The road to human spiritual transformation lies before us, and many have found that developing good self-pacing skills is at the center of a successful approach. It means we are well on the way to self-sufficiency in our spiritual endeavors. Responsible use of practices with self-pacing is the key to sustaining forward progress in the enlightenment process. It means we can do it ourselves. Once we know that, then there is no stopping us.

Teaching

Everyone is able to teach yoga from their own level of experience. Anyone who has become grounded in deep meditation, spinal breathing, etc., to whatever level, can pass that experience on to others. The *AYP writings* are sufficiently detailed so anyone can take their direct experience and pass it on, using the writings as an aid and a stimulus. So we should all feel free to do that to the degree we are comfortable, within our own inner silence. This is beneficial to both the teacher and the student. The teacher always learns at least as much as the student.

There have been reservations expressed over the years on the hazards of people teaching yoga beyond their level of attainment. Indeed, this is a hazard with any teacher, even the advanced ones who may be the ones expressing the concern. To hold everyone back for the sake of this concern is unrealistic. A title or a certification does not guarantee complete, integrated teaching. Most often, such credentials are certifications of a sectarian approach, which is much better than no teachings, but still quite limited.

What we really need is many more people rising independently in inner silence and divine ecstasy from within, and sharing that in daily life by all means that suit the situation and culture. As we move forward in this new era, the teachings will come from within like that, much more than from external systems. External systems will no longer be the primary source of knowledge. They will only be for facilitating the flow of *stillness in action* coming from within.

If we are sharing a pragmatic integration of knowledge based on the direct experience happening within ourselves, then that will be title and certification enough to teach anyone. If we keep coming back to the fundamental principles and practices inherent in the human nervous system, how can we go wrong? That is the reason why the *AYP writings* are being put out in public view. Not to create a following, a movement, or an organization. Not to stand as a monolithic body of teachings either. But to be a resource that can be woven into daily considerations of spiritual transformation in many ways – a touchstone of truth that can help anyone become a beacon of light to themselves and to many others. The AYP teachings do not come from any specific lineage. They come from the broad (and often ancient) multi-cultural knowledge of humankind. And, most importantly, from verifications of the practices in the present through direct experience in the human nervous system.

As open source teachings like the *AYP writings* come much more into the public awareness, more *horizontal transmission* of knowledge will be occurring according to the direct experience of steadily increasing numbers of practitioners around the world who continue to share what they have learned through word of mouth. This kind of spiritual knowledge transmission has also been called *peer-to-peer*. Due to its inherent non-hierarchal nature, this style of knowledge transmission avoids many of the pitfalls found in hierarchal systems where the abuse of power over others is commonplace. The horizontal peer-to-peer structure is "candles lighting candles until all candles are lit." This is possible with the rise of real spiritual progress in many practitioners. It is not only the transmission of ideas. It is also the transmission of spiritual energy that quickens the process of human spiritual transformation in everyone. Before now, this has not been possible. With the rapid rise of consciousness around the world, this new mode of teaching is taking hold – the direct transmission of knowledge and spiritual energy, which is *stillness in action.*

In terms of practices, it is a step-by-step process of inspiring bhakti (spiritual desire), and then providing the tools for the cultivation of inner silence and ecstatic conductivity in every individual.

Those who have traveled far along the path are to be reminded that everyone must travel from where they are using the most effective methods. There is a tendency for those who are advanced in spiritual progress to teach the destination (their present condition) as being the path. This can lead students to engage in what we call *non-relational self-inquiry* into the non-dual nature of existence. That is, inquiry in the mind and not in stillness, which is largely fruitless and can be psychologically harmful. With the rise of inner silence (the witness), *relational self-inquiry* becomes possible. So the first priority is the cultivation of inner silence. In the AYP approach, this is accomplished with deep meditation and related means.

The same is also true in teaching about our relationship with karma, the events occurring around us, and with the times we will experience pain in our life. There will be pain, but it can be borne without suffering. But not by only being told that this is so. It is with the rise of inner silence (the witness) that we can transcend suffering that comes with the identification of the mind with thinking, feelings and our perception of the world around us. As we become free from identification with the objects of perception, no matter how glorious or painful they may be, we can share our freedom with others, and we can also share the means for others to be free within themselves. It is in all of us.

As time goes on, many illuminated practitioners will become more visible, along with the supporting written teachings. Writings that are true, and flexible in their application, will have a long shelf life, and will not wear out. In time, the application of methods and the experiences of practitioners around the world will naturally expand to encompass all eight limbs of yoga.

Those who are engaged in *self-directed integrated practices* are on the leading edge. From this, the field of yoga will become increasingly more centered on fostering individual self-sufficiency in cultivating the overall process of human spiritual transformation. To the extent enlightenment has been occurring in the world over the centuries, it has always been based on individual self-sufficiency.

Our schools and institutions for higher learning will find an expanding role in this, because the people will be noticing it occurring around them, and demanding the necessary education. The teaching of integrated spiritual practices will be happening in yoga studios, retreat centers, trade schools and universities across the land. But first, it will be happening in the homes of practitioners everywhere, as a vast and diverse network expands outward until everyone has been touched.

These days, spiritual transformation is rising in millions. It is something new that has been steadily accelerating over the past century, an emergence of yoga and spiritual practices on a vast scale – it is a global phenomenon. In this highly energized situation, just a little bit of the right information will go a long way. Individual desire/bhakti and daily practice will take care of the rest.

So, let us all do what our inner silence moves us to do in our practices and our teaching. And, by all means, have fun while doing it!

Practices for Our Children

It is natural to want to share our spiritual knowledge with our children. We may especially want to share deep meditation with them. There can be great benefits. How we go about sharing practices will depend on the age of our children.

Easy *I AM* deep meditation can be practiced upon reaching 12-13 years of age. The suggestion is to start out with 10 minutes maximum per twice-daily sitting. If there is an undesirable result, too much purification, then less time, or none, should be used until a year or two later, and then try again. Too much purification is usually noticeable as irritability and/or dullness in daily activity. Of course, with teenagers and new hormones flowing, that may be happening anyway. Daily meditation in the right dosage can be a help.

Excessive purification can happen if the nervous system is very sensitive to meditation, which indicates a high spiritual sensitivity – a good thing, but it should be handled carefully using the principles of self-pacing.

Assuming all is going smoothly, once age 18 is reached, the time of meditation can be inched up 5 minutes at a time over several months to 20 minutes, as comfortable. By this time, the young practitioner will have an established interest, or not, depending on individual karma and desire. We should not force it. At this stage, it will be as much the inner condition of the young practitioner that will determine the path as what the parent or teacher can offer. Many children will drop meditation for a variety of reasons. But the seed is planted. The rest will be up to individual desire in relation to the flow of nature and karma. This is true for all of us, yes? The good news is that the spiritual tide is rising everywhere. Everyone is becoming more attuned to their inner transformation. So, any seeds that are planted these days are certain to germinate and grow to full blossom – if not here and now, then somewhere along the glimmering road of this life, or perhaps the next one. Our gift will not be wasted.

Light alternate nostril breathing (nadi shodana pranayama) can be used by teenagers before meditation for 5 minutes, or so. It is a common practice that can be learned almost anywhere – it is covered in the *AYP Easy Lessons* book. Alternate nostril breathing can also be used in short sessions by pre-teens (without meditation) if emotions need some soothing influence. Alternate nostril breathing of 5-10 minutes several times per day can be helpful for hyperactive children. If alternate nostril breathing is not comfortable, then simple slow deep breathing through both nostrils can be used instead.

At age 18, the alternate nostril breathing (or slow deep breathing) can be replaced with spinal breathing pranayama, inching the time up as appropriate. Advanced pranayama-related methods, mudras and bandhas, are for expanding the sexual function upward into higher manifestation in the nervous system, and that is why techniques beyond easy deep meditation and light alternate nostril or deep breathing should not be used before or during puberty. Spiritual transformation in the nervous system, the expansion of neurobiological functioning to express divine ecstasy, is like a second puberty in many respects. One puberty at a time is enough!

For some young adults, taking on a full range of practices may be delayed far beyond 18 years old. For others sooner may be okay. Everyone is different, and we should use our best judgment in making suggestions on this. Once spinal breathing pranayama and deep meditation are progressive and stable, then going step-by-step through the full range of practices can be undertaken according to one's desire (bhakti) and capacity (self-pacing). This is the adult stage, of course.

Light yoga postures (asanas) can be undertaken, using good common sense, at any age. Once sitting practice/meditation is begun, then asanas can be done right before that. Asanas can be learned almost anywhere these days, with children's classes becoming quite common. The *AYP writings* include an *asana starter kit*, which can be helpful for getting started with an easy routine of postures at home.

Regarding our youngest children, sharing our own rising inner silence in the form of overflowing loving service is the ideal yoga for them. They will benefit greatly, and be ready for practices when the time comes, according to their own inclinations. Obviously, we cannot dictate what another's inclinations will be – even our own children's.

Everyone has their own journey to make. We can help a lot, but we can't do it all for them. Let's be careful not to hem our children into a practice routine that is not natural for them. Remember, it is their inner silence that will ultimately determine their path more than anything else.

One thing is for sure. The more we can progress in our own practices, the better it will be for our loved ones. That is how we can stimulate inner silence in everyone.

Open Source Research – Road to the Future

Everyone who engages in self-directed spiritual practices is a researcher in consciousness. In the past, this has been a lonely profession, reserved for the few, often done in secret, with little shared with the general population. For this reason, much of spiritual knowledge has been called arcane and esoteric. Perhaps there were good reasons. Knowledge was not very portable in centuries past, and there was much superstition surrounding the process of human spiritual transformation. Even those who spoke clearly about it (like Patanjali) did not find a large audience. It is only through the centuries that recorded knowledge on spiritual practices has come to be utilized more widely.

In our time, we have a great opportunity. This is the information age, and we are in the midst of an explosion of applied knowledge in all fields of human endeavor. It is happening in the field of human spiritual transformation also.

Now we have open access to many more practices, and are in the process of integrating and applying the means that directly cultivate purification and opening within us on an accelerated scale. The eight limbs of yoga are no longer only a list of the possibilities and interrelationships of practices and experiences, but are also a list which we can apply using real resources for transformation. We are expanding from the philosophical into the practical, and every day is a learning experience by which we can make adjustments in practices leading to ever more knowledge of ourselves.

The journey we each are on is our research, and it should be shared. In this way, we can find out what we have in common in our development and what may be divergent from the norm. In fact, we are finding the divergences to be far less than have been believed. The divergences have been mostly man-made. The human nervous system is the same everywhere, and its capabilities for purification and opening to divine experience are also the same.

So what do we not have in common? Perhaps our culture and religion, and the variations in methods that have been handed down to us. But, in the end, we are all working on the same project, no matter where we have come from or what tools we are using. The eight limbs cover the full range, and if we are focused in one limb, we will surely find the others through the connectedness of yoga, alive within us.

By practicing, self-pacing, documenting and open sharing, the truth will continue to emerge in modern times. This is the road to the future. It is in our hands to sustain the advance of *applied spiritual science* for all time.

We should continue to look back enough into the ancient recorded knowledge so we can continue to move forward to more efficient applications of knowledge. But we should not look back thinking that the ancients knew more than we can know. We want to stand on their great shoulders to reach higher still, manifesting the truth of ancient knowledge in our experience in the present. And we are.

There are plenty of spiritual pioneers emerging these days who are marching forward with the systematic application of spiritual practices in ways that have not been tried before. Modern institutions of research and higher learning will catch on eventually, and then lead the way in thoroughly researching the methods of human spiritual transformation, supported by an ever-growing segment of the population engaged in daily practices.

Why will the institutions eventually take the lead? Because there are great issues of the public welfare at stake – the health, well-being and happiness of all the nations and cultures of the world. As we unfold the full potential of the individual, so too will we unfold the full potential of societies everywhere around the world. Just as information technologies have changed life on earth, so too will spiritual technologies enhance the quality of life everywhere. This is why the large institutions will become deeply involved in uncovering the specific mechanisms of human spiritual transformation, and the means for optimizing them on every level.

As in all other fields of human endeavor, ongoing research and development for the practical application of spiritual knowledge will carry us to a quality of life we can scarcely imagine today.

It is all contained in seed form in the eight limbs of yoga, which are a reflection of what is waiting to be unfolded in each of us. Now we are bringing our full potential to fruition, and everyone will share in this.

This will not be knowledge based on the charismatic personalities that have come and gone in every generation. Rather, it will be knowledge that is recorded and constantly evolving to more efficient applications, which can be verified and practically utilized by everyone on the earth.

Chapter 4 – The Rise of Enlightenment

Since ancient times, it has been known that human spiritual experience includes two components – stillness and ecstasy. Various terminologies are used in cultures around the world to designate these fundamental constituents of human spiritual transformation. Whether we are talking about Shiva and Kundalini/Shakti, God the Father and the Holy Spirit, Tao and Chi, or other terms, we are always talking about the same thing – the experience of purification and opening in the nervous system, which is the doorway to the divine found in all of humanity.

In time, and with an effective integration of spiritual practices spanning the full range of the eight limbs of yoga, the duality of our experience evolves to become the non-dual unity of divine experience, or *stillness in action*. It is then that we know what we have been all along – *Oneness*.

Along the way we will pass by milestones that indicate the emergence of stillness, the rise of ecstatic conductivity, and the merging of these two.

Enlightenment Milestones

The destination of our life is *enlightenment*. What is enlightenment? A state of balanced union between our two natures: pure bliss consciousness, and our involvement as sentient beings on this physical earth. That is also the definition of yoga, and the destination of all religion too.

The evolution of experience is a personal journey, but it has a certain recognizable pattern, with three identifiable stages:

- The rise of abiding inner silence.
- The rise of ecstatic conductivity and radiance.
- The joining of these into outpouring divine love and unity.

The rise of inner silence (samadhi) comes from daily deep meditation. It is experienced as an increasingly steady state of peace, happiness and bliss. Most of all, it is experienced as an inner stability that is not shaken by any outer experience – the *witness*. Inner silence is the foundation for further experiences that are facilitated by additional yoga practices that awaken the silence of pure bliss consciousness to a dynamic state in our nervous system.

The rise of ecstatic experience (kundalini) in the body and surroundings comes from an awakening of the life force in the body and a gradual refinement of sensory perception. Through pranayama (breathing methods), mudras, bandhas, tantric sexual techniques and other means, inner purification and opening is enhanced so the senses are opened in an inward direction (pratyahara), enabling us to perceive the ecstatic energies coursing within and around us. In this way our attention and sense of self are drawn inward, and eventually radiated outward, giving us a new perspective on the world around us.

At the same time, silence begins to move within us, facilitated by the radiant nature of ecstatic energy, and this creates a new and captivating kind of experience. During this stage, appreciation for the divine flow of life is naturally heightened, leading to increased desire to enter and merge with the deepening sensory experience. One surrenders to the process as it advances, and this accelerates it.

The second stage is like falling into an endless abyss of ecstasy. We function in the world with increasing joy as our attention becomes absorbed in the ever-present living beauty moving beneath the surface of all things. For us, the boundaries are dissolving.

As our attention comes to reside naturally in the omnipresent, undulating blissful silence in all things, we become that ever-present harmony. We find our own *Self* to be the essence of all things. This is the experience of unity, union, enlightenment. The world does not disappear. It becomes transparent and radiant. Boundaries become like veils, thinly covering the essence of life, which we have come to know as an expression of our own nature. We realize through direct perception that we are the ocean upon which the waves of life are playing.

In this condition, can we still act in the world? Yes, but our motives are different than before when we could only see ourselves as separate. We now act in the interest of a broader *Self*. In doing so, we may seem to become selfless. The truth is that we always are acting for our own self-interest. But our *Self* has become transcendent and universal, so our interest is for the whole of humanity, and for the whole of life. We no longer see the world as an illusion of separate things that we may either crave or fear. We see it for what it is, an endless flow of divine being, and we find ourselves in the position to help others open themselves to a natural awareness of things as they are also. It is life in freedom begetting more life in freedom. It is the destiny of every person, and of all humanity.

From the beginning of engaging in our practices (and perhaps even before), we may experience shades of any of the three stages mentioned above, depending on the dynamics of our unique purification process. We may experience elements of all three stages at the same time. Over time, we come to recognize the telltale experiences as milestones on the way to enlightenment – some inner silence, some inner ecstatic flow, a sense of *Oneness* with others and our environment. There will be many more sub-milestones we notice as we move along. The milestones are useful to keep us going, to keep us inspired and regular in our daily practices.

The milestones are not so useful for proclaiming, "Today I am here along the road to enlightenment."

Indeed, we may well be, but it will only be significant when we have gone past there and our experience has become permanent, unspectacular and little noticed. When the experience becomes natural and normal it becomes real, part of our everyday life, and no longer a spectacle in the mind, which is prone to flights of fancy.

Enlightenment is not a spectacle. It is life as we are meant to live it – liberation is quite ordinary. The milestones will be dissolved in the journey. Ultimately, enlightenment is not so much about the milestones. It is about enjoying becoming and being that which we always have been.

If we are making a long car trip, do we spend all our time marveling at the scenery along the way? Maybe to some degree, but, if we are really interested in arriving at our destination, it will not be to the point of interrupting our journey. We can enjoy the scenery along the way without stopping for too long, forgetting what we are doing on the road – traveling home.

We may be inclined to notice the particulars of our journey for the benefit of others. After all, everyone emanates from the same divine consciousness as we do, so we are naturally concerned that all should have a safe and speedy ride.

Jesus said, "Do unto others as you would have them do unto you."

The truth is that all others are us, so this is not only good moral advice, it is good practical advice. Experientially, we come to know that others are our own *Self*, as our inner doors are opened to the divine realms within.

How long does the journey take? It depends mainly on us – on our past actions that have produced the obstructions lodged deep in our nervous system, and on what we do from now on. We can't change the past. But we can do much in the present that will shape our future. No one else can make the choice but us. If we take up yoga practices with sincere devotion, there will be a new direction in our life. Once we have committed ourselves unswervingly to the path, it is only a matter of time. Then we see it is not so much about the final destination. It is about experiencing increasing joy each day, each month, and each year. This is a path of bliss, a path of pleasure, as we naturally unfold from within. We can get on the path today and begin to enjoy the ride immediately. We will get to the end, bye and bye.

The Divine Marriage

Once our desire inspires us to make a direct approach to the process of human spiritual transformation, applying the means for cultivating abiding inner silence will be the first step. It is deep meditation. As inner silence begins to come up, a range of additional practices can be added, leading to the expansion of stillness in daily activity, much the way a pump will greatly expand the supply of water once the pump has been primed.

Some of the practices we add to deep meditation will stimulate the rise of ecstatic conductivity in the nervous system.

Ecstatic conductivity is cultivated with different kinds of practices than are used for the cultivation of inner silence. Inner silence relies on the practice of deep meditation, and is then expanded through samyama. Ecstatic conductivity is cultivated with spinal breathing pranayama, asanas, mudras, bandhas, and tantric sexual methods. These are different classes of practice altogether.

Practices related to the cultivation of ecstatic conductivity enhance both deep meditation and samyama. This is because they loosen the subtle neurobiology. Pranayama is especially effective for this, and the loosening is further facilitated with asanas, mudras, bandhas and tantric methods. These methods are energy-related, and cultivate the soil of the nervous system to make it a better vehicle for inner silence, or pure bliss consciousness.

So here we have the beginning of the relationship of inner silence and ecstasy. The movement of subtle energy in the body (*prana*) and its unmistakable ecstatic quality is facilitated by the rise of inner silence. At the same time, the rise of inner silence is facilitated by the movement of inner ecstatic energy. Each enables the other!

Some practices straddle the divide between inner silence and ecstasy, working both sides of the fence, so to speak. The methods of samyama, self-inquiry and the rising urge to engage in more service in life without an agenda (*karma yoga*) are in this category.

As we release a natural intention, an inquiry or an action in silence, we are stimulating stillness to move. To the extent we have ecstatic conductivity present, that movement of stillness will take on the quality of ecstasy, while at the same time retaining the quality of bliss, which is an inherent characteristic of inner silence. The result is moving ecstatic bliss, which is the fuel of divine expression in the world. Over time, stillness and ecstasy become intimately intertwined in all that we do, and this is the marriage.

With the marriage of inner silence and ecstasy, a new dynamic is born. We could call it *ecstatic bliss*, but that hardly describes it. We sometimes use the phrase *abiding inner silence, ecstatic bliss and outpouring divine love*. This more fully captures the dynamic that is occurring. There is stillness – *abiding inner silence*. There is an inner radiance that contains the qualities of both pure bliss consciousness and ecstatic conductivity – *ecstatic bliss*. And there is movement outward as the flow of radiance seeks to express itself through the nervous system – *outpouring divine love*, which produces a unifying influence within and around us – *Oneness*.

From the point of view of the practitioner, we find a lot of pleasure in this on many levels. It is physical and psychological pleasure. The outflow is luminous and the world becomes luminous as well. Not that the nature of the world has changed, but we have changed in the way we see it and operate in it. We see it for what it really is – an infinite flow of energy that is in a constant joyous dance. The negative interpretations that predominate in so much of human life are seen in an entirely different light. The foibles of mind are seen to be outrageous!

So what do we do when we come to see the world in this way? Do we run away and hide out in a cave? No way. Surely there are ways to help everyone to see what we see. From within ourselves we are moved to do that – to help in whatever way we can. It is an outpouring, an outpouring of divine love.

This third element, the outpouring, that comes from the merging of our inner silence and ecstatic conductivity is the proverbial child of enlightenment. It has been called *Christ, savior, jivan mukti (liberated soul)*. It is not we in the personal egoic sense who become this. It is the divine flowing through us that is this birth, this outpouring, and we become consciously dissolved in *It*, surrendered to *It*, becoming *It*.

Our activities in daily life play an important role in cultivating and stabilizing this divine flow. The essence of enlightenment is active surrender, doing and letting go. If we set up the initial conditions of inner silence and ecstatic conductivity with our practices, and then engage fully in life, the merging and divine birth will occur.

Then we will find ourselves flying on the wings of ecstatic bliss in everything we do. And we will be surrounded by wonderful miraculous happenings. All of nature rushes to support a divine outpouring. Once the divine pump has been primed, the flow increases without limit. By learning to do in practices and in life, and let go, we are able to unleash infinite good in the world.

Prudent application of the eight limbs of yoga brings us naturally to this permanent condition of happiness and evolutionary divine presence. Then we find that we have become unending *stillness in action*, and every moment of our life is an expression of pure joy.

The guru is in you.

Further Reading and Support

Yogani is an American spiritual scientist who, for more than thirty years, has been integrating ancient techniques from around the world which cultivate human spiritual transformation. The approach he has developed is non-sectarian, and open to all. In the order published, his books include:

Advanced Yoga Practices – Easy Lessons for Ecstatic Living
A large user-friendly textbook providing 240 detailed lessons on the AYP integrated system of yoga practices.

The Secrets of Wilder – A Novel
The story of young Americans discovering and utilizing actual secret practices leading to human spiritual transformation.

The AYP Enlightenment Series
Easy-to-read instruction books on yoga practices, including:

- *Deep Meditation – Pathway to Personal Freedom*
- *Spinal Breathing Pranayama – Journey to Inner Space*
- *Tantra – Discovering the Power of Pre-Orgasmic Sex*
- *Asanas, Mudras and Bandhas – Awakening Ecstatic Kundalini*
- *Samyama – Cultivating Stillness in Action, Siddhis and Miracles*
- *Diet, Shatkarmas and Amaroli – Yogic Nutrition and Cleansing for Health and Spirit*
- *Self Inquiry – Dawn of the Witness and the End of Suffering*
- *Bhakti and Karma Yoga – The Science of Devotion and Liberation Through Action*
- *Eight Limbs of Yoga – The Structure and Pacing of Self-Directed Spiritual Practice*

For up-to-date information on the writings of Yogani, and for the free *AYP Support Forums*, please visit:

www.advancedyogapractices.com

CPSIA information can be obtained at www.ICGtesting.com
Printed in the USA

265828BV00001B/104/P